The Medellin Wellness Protocol

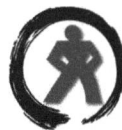

SUPER-A BOOKS

The Medellin Wellness Protocol

The Five Fundamental Factors to Strengthen your Immune System

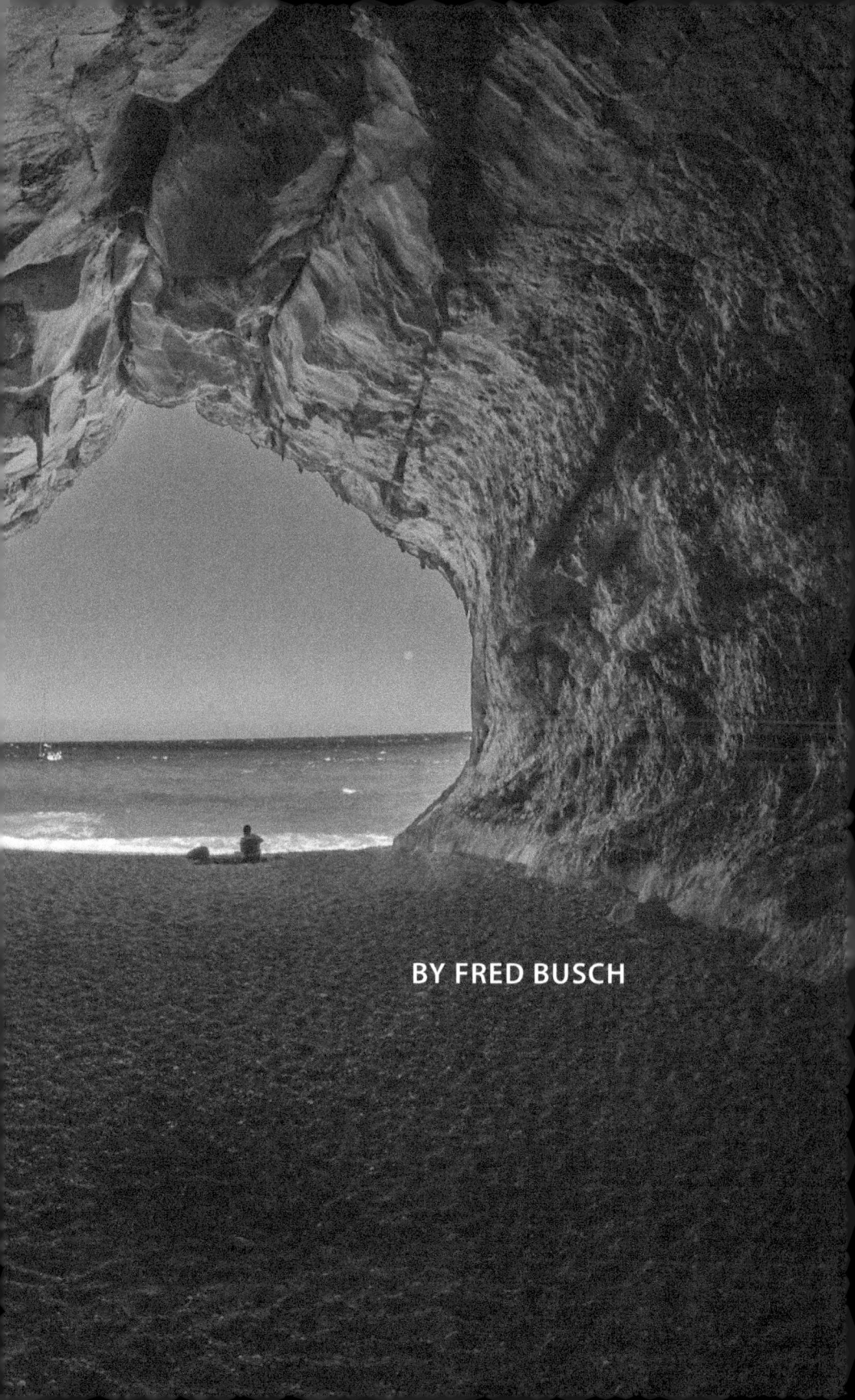

BY FRED BUSCH

First published in 2021 by Super-A Books

Copyright © Fred Busch

The right of Fred Busch to be identified as the author of this work has been asserted in accordance with the Copyright, Designs and Patents Act, 1988.

ISBN: 978-1-8383579-0-0

A CIP catalogue record for this book is available from The British Library

Design by Carnegie Book Production

Super-A Books is an imprint of Libri Publishing

Super-A Books
Brunel House
Volunteer Way
Faringdon
Oxfordshire
SN7 7YR

Tel: +44 (0)845 873 3837

www.libripublishing.co.uk

CONTENTS

Introduction from the Author

The health and wellbeing of the human population is suffering under the weight of several influences. These influences such as diet, exercise, mental programming, sleep deprivation and toxic exposure have a debilitating effect on the immune system. Our immune system is central to our health and wellbeing and this book will guide the reader through the fundamental factors everyone needs to learn and employ to have a strong immune system, prevent disease and reverse health conditions.

Stated simply, the human immune system is located throughout the body and found inside the body's drainage system known as the lymphatic system. The essential function of our immune system is to dispatch intelligent cells to identify and destroy foreign invaders such as germs, bacteria and viruses that seek to damage and sicken our bodies.

A healthy body will efficiently and effectively identify and destroy these potentially harmful entities before they cause illness and disease. An unhealthy body with an impaired immune system will be overwhelmed and defeated by these invaders causing sickness, disease and potential death.

It is extremely important to remember that the state of your immune system is not static.

In other words, a compromised immune system does not need to be a permanent condition and can be vastly improved with modifications in diet and lifestyle. Thus, you have control over your health because you can strengthen your immune system.

The Five Fundamental Factors of the Medellin Wellness Protocol will provide the roadmap that will help you achieve that goal.

It is my hope that by reading this book and doing the simple steps required of you, you will attain your goals of a greater quality of life in all dimensions.

Yours in light and awareness,

Fred Busch

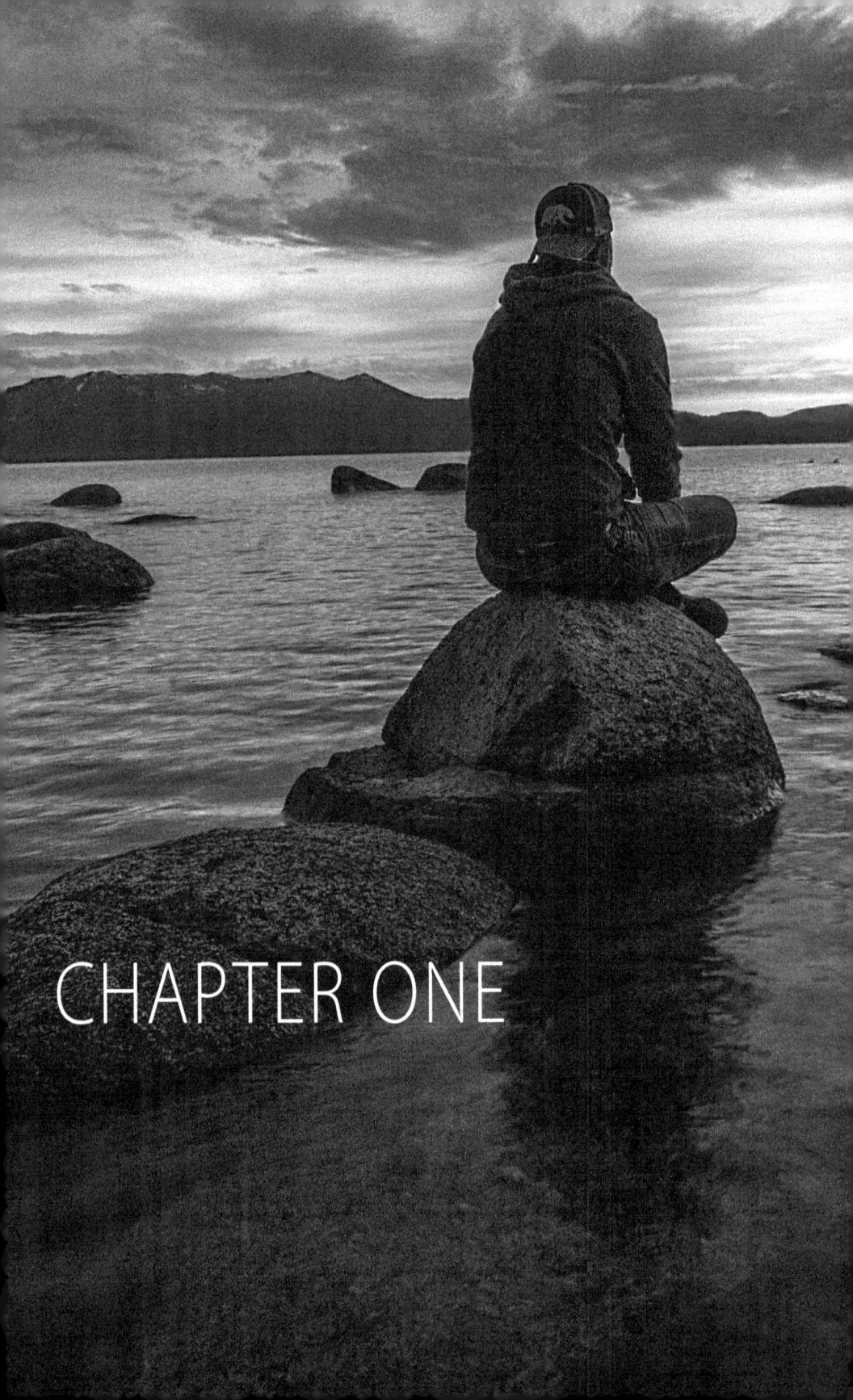

CHAPTER ONE

Strengthening the Immune System and Resisting Pandemics

The human immune system is capable of wonderful things even beyond our comprehension. When we are confronted by viruses, even pandemics, the only factor that all experts and the medical scientists agree is most determinative to people's outcome is the immune system. That a compromised immune system will lead to potential negative outcomes for individuals under threat of disease is now common knowledge. But many people speak of the immune system without understanding really what it is.

WHAT IS THE IMMUNE SYSTEM AND HOW DO WE STRENGTHEN IT?

The immune system is called a system and so it may be easy to think of it like the other systems of the body as classified in human anatomy. This would not be an accurate picture however because the other 'systems' of the body have structures and defined locations that can be isolated and identified.

The cardiovascular system, for example, is made of the heart and blood vessels. The respiratory system is made of lungs and pulmonary arteries that can be easily located and even removed or acted upon surgically.

The immune system however is qualitatively different and must be appreciated on its own terms so that it can be understood how exactly to make it work better. The human immune system is located throughout the entire body and found inside the body's drainage network known as the lymphatic system.

The immune system is not one singular system with structure and location but rather a hive of intelligent cells that are dispatched by the overall intelligence of the body to identify, mark, then destroy any entity that is not welcome. The immune system is a constellation of intelligence-guided intercommunicating cells which are able to identify and then neutralize the many different foreign invaders that can find their way into the vital domain.

This may be the first time you have heard the word intelligence associated so strongly with discussion of the immune system but it will soon be clear.

All cells in our body, and in particular immune system cells, have a very specific job description and this job requires perfect functioning in order to prevail. A half-operative immune cell will likely not be able to finish its job and may leave the foreign invader able to continue its course.

While this may be repetitive to some who are well studied, there can be no discussing the immune system without a formal introduction to the lymphatic system because #1 the immune system lives in the lymphatic system, and #2 the environment of the lymphatic system and its potential stagnation completely determines the functional capacity of the immune cells.

The lymphatic system is the waste removal system of the body and runs throughout the body in a series of lymph vessels and nodes which collect the waste drained from the interstitial fluid. These wastes are acidic in nature and the lymph system is designed to bring the waste materials to the kidneys for elimination. Any compromising of the lymphatic system's ability to eliminate waste will result in acidic waste buildup in the fluids which house the immune system.

The immune system's cells are floating in the river of lymphatic fluid throughout the body as well as in glands where they are produced, such as the Thymus.

The lymphatic fluid can be either acidic or alkaline depending on the person's lifestyle and diet and depending on whether there is sufficient elimination of cellular waste. If the lymph fluids are not able to drain properly due to problems with elimination then the acidic waste begins to build up in the lymph system, including in the various lymph nodes, causing swelling and hardness in otherwise supple and non-swollen tissue. When the buildup of acids persists in the lymph fluid, whatever is inside the lymph fluid is going to be 'burned' or damaged by the acids of cellular and metabolic wastes that have not been eliminated and instead keep increasing in concentration over time.

When an immune system cell is burned by the lymphatic fluid's acidic constituents (wastes of cell metabolism) then the immune cells are no longer able to function at 100% capacity.

Returning to the idea of intelligence and immune cells now we can appreciate that an immune cell that is caught stagnated in an acidic (burning) fluid will be damaged and this acts as a kind of damage to the cell's intelligence, which is to say the ability to make decisions and execute the challenging action of neutralizing foreign entities.

Here is a vitally important and yet missing link of information to this subject that is not well understood even by those who are promoting the immune system as the only answer:

All viruses including the class of coronaviruses are proteins. These proteins are foreign to the body and as a result the body immediately begins a process of elimination which comes in the form of mucus that can then accumulate in places like the sinuses or lungs. Those without a strong capacity for elimination of mucus from the lungs are those who are not as well equipped to recover easily from the detoxification process initiated by the virus-protein.

So in many ways the important subject is our immune system and its ability to fend off invaders and neutralize proteins, but the other aspect of a healthy immune system is a well-operating lymphatic system so that the immune cells can always be 100% capacitized and not compromised. When the detox process begins, due to exposure to any virus, the key is that the eliminative lymphatic channels open and are able to eliminate the waste materials effectively. This allows the process of recovery from the viral detoxification event to be fast and relatively painless.

IS THE STATE OF YOUR IMMUNE SYSTEM SOMETHING THAT IS STATIC?

Once you are designated as a member of an at-risk group does that mean that there is nothing you can do? Not at all! The immune system's intelligence and functioning can be reactivated and reinvigorated by providing a specific environment here in this work.

The Five Fundamental Factors outlined in the Medellin Wellness Protocol address all the factors that are responsible for

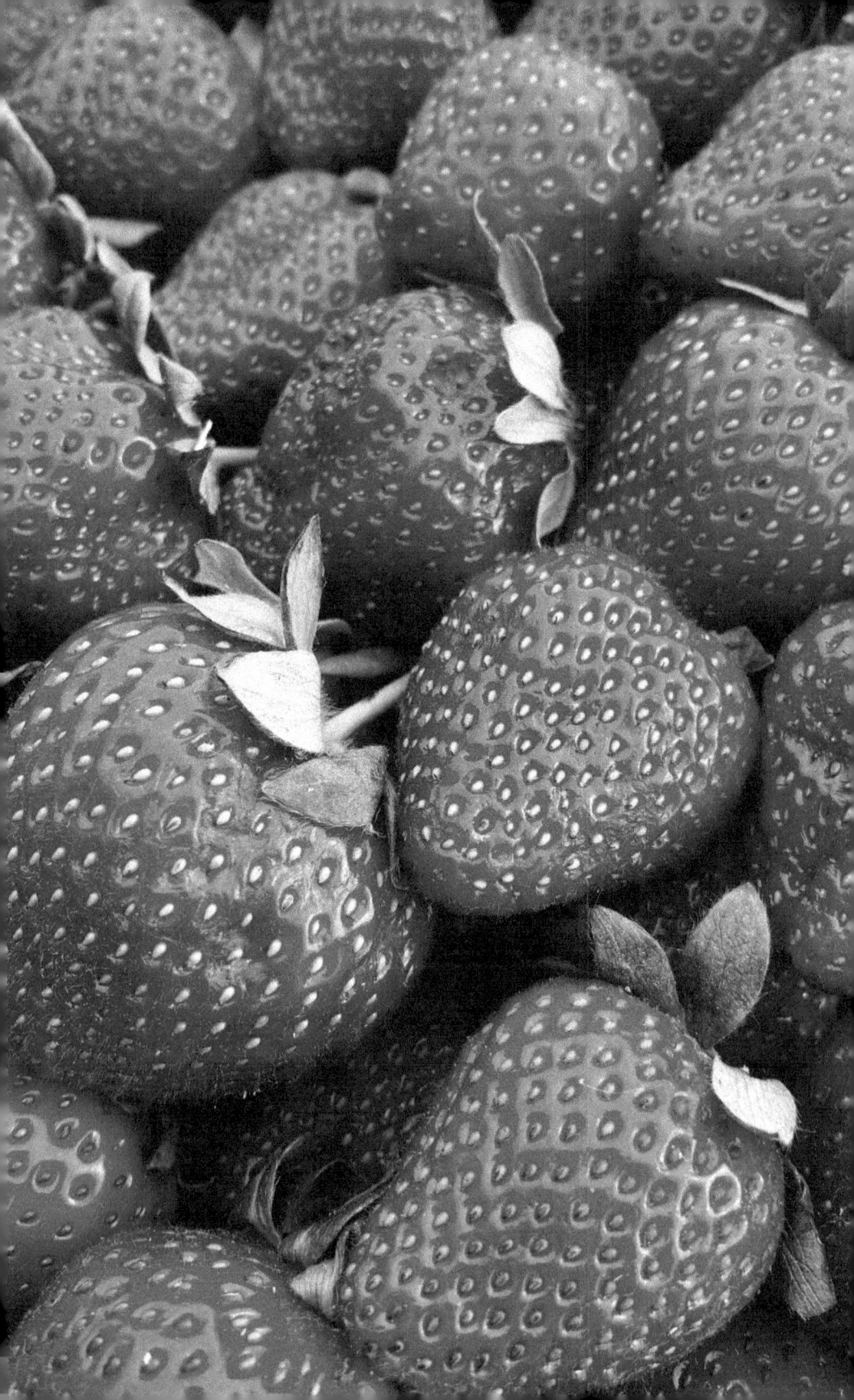

compromising your immune system, and once these causes are addressed and removed the immune system can begin to function as it was designed.

In fact these Five Fundamental Factors are each in their own right responsible for supporting immune system health.

HOW DO WE EAT?

Elimination of mucus from the body is of the highest priority for any person involved in any virus-initiated or detox process. Due to their hydrating, energizing, alkalizing, astringing, electromagnetically charged nature, only fruits can assist the body with this process and this is why it is the number one recommended food for immune system health.

HOW DO WE EXERCISE?

Depending on the health and energy levels of a person, a moderate amount of daily exercise is highly valuable for moving lymph fluids and assisting elimination while stimulating the healthy action of immune systems cells.

HOW DO WE USE OUR MIND?

The mind is central to our experience of reality. Additionally each thought we think has a corresponding reaction in the chemistry of our body. Negative or self-limiting patterns of thinking can literally suppress the immune system while a positive and intentional use of the mind can turn on the engines of immune capacity through the parasympathetic nervous system.

HOW DO WE REST?

Rest and relaxation is something everybody intuitively understands is related to immune system health. Sleep deprivation and over stimulation in daily life go together and will always result in lower immune system functioning. Learning how to rest well and sleep well is key!

HOW DO WE LIVE MORE ORGANICALLY?

Many people are overloading their immune system through continual exposure to toxins that are so common that they are not even recognized as a threat. Toxic poisons entering our system in the form or food or drink or household chemicals tend to devastate the immune system for both reasons outlined above.

As you are about to discover when you put these Five Fundamental Factors together in your life you will begin to feel propelled by a positive feedback cycle that will empower your immune health to fight any disease that comes your way.

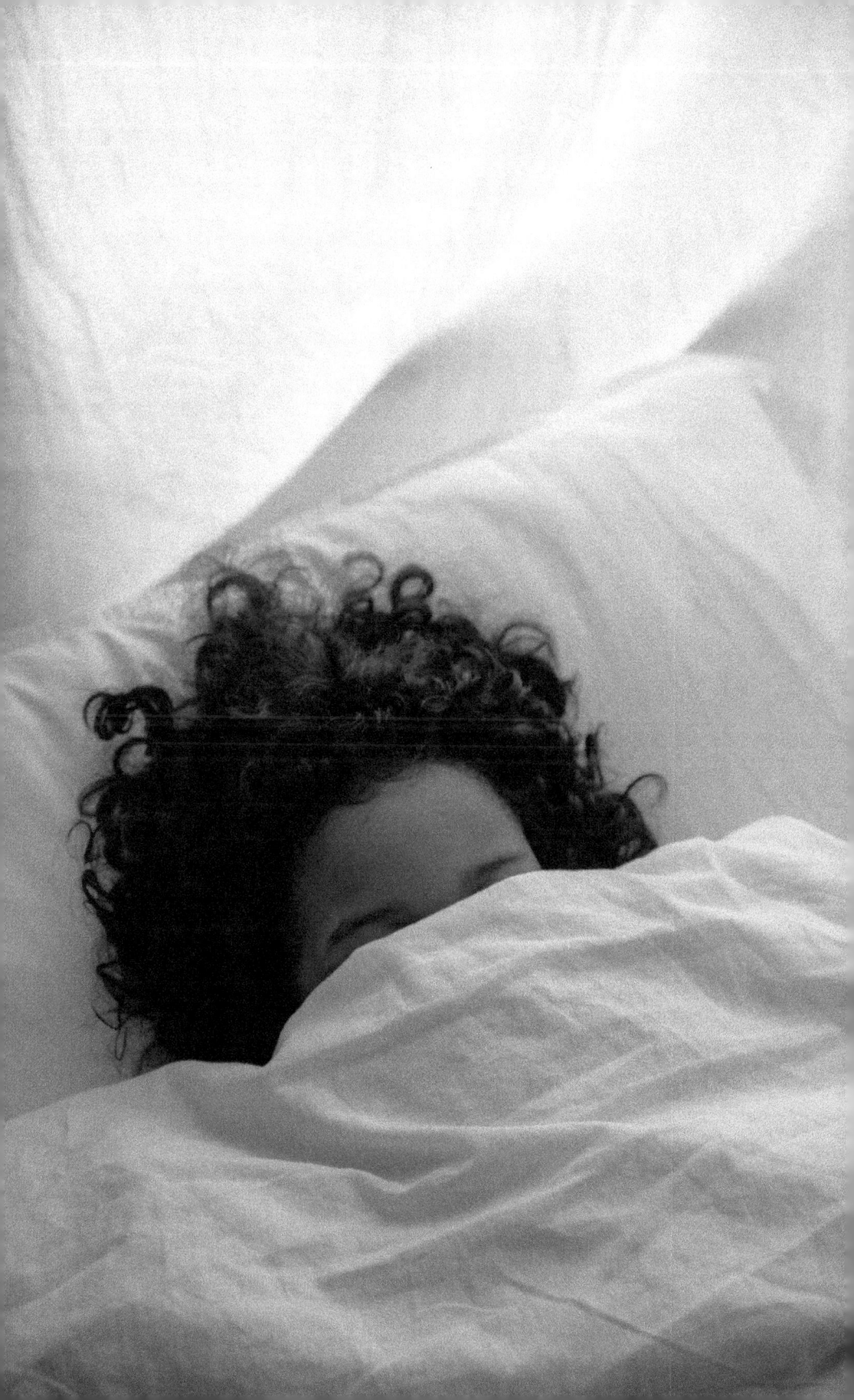

CHAPTER 2

Refocusing the Lens

There are several reasons why many doctors are often unable to provide the most effective and appropriate solution for their patients. One primary reason for this is that medical doctors are focused on the symptoms rather than the causes of any given situation. Another reason is that doctors have become very specialized. Specialists are by design unable to see the holistic bigger picture. Also specialists are not able to see factors that are not related to their field which may very likely be affecting the condition. A specialist doctor's perspective on a person's health issue is limited to the narrow focus area.

This is a fundamental mistake that is creating confusion about wellness since many experts are so specialized that nobody really understands the fact that more than one variable is at play in causing the condition. As a result of this specialization the doctors are only addressing one variable of what is a multivariable equation. This is a very dubious process that is not ideal since humans are not simply separated organ systems.

The medical professionals we trust to regain or maintain our health are looking only through the lens of their own field of expertise and have little ability to focus on overall wellness.

Why are the rates of diseases and conditions like diabetes, heart disease, ulcers, esophageal reflux, poor mental health, chronic pain and the like so high? How is this possible when the access to knowledge and ability to reach the masses through media is so powerful?

One rather obvious answer is that all too frequently, our health professionals are focusing only on the narrow problem before them and not the overall 'big picture' needed for true wellness.

An example of this is the doctor who gives medications before talking about lifestyle factors.

This is also true in the non-medical world of specialists in wellness. For example a talented personal trainer who coaches the physical body well is likely ignoring the mind and giving incorrect nutritional advice. The classically trained nutritionists of today are not trained in accurate nutritional science and also ignore the importance of exercise and the mind. Mental health professionals working with the mind ignore the important if not causative relationship between nutrition, exercise and the mind.

And the list goes on of experts who work in their field without realizing that their field represents only one of the factors or variables needed to attain good mental and physical health.

THE MULTIDIMENSIONAL APPROACH

A multidimensional approach must be taken to achieve the goal we all seek – good health and happiness. It is simply not enough to only focus on the body, or the mind, or the spirit, or nutrition. Whether it is the overspecialization of the medical field or the divergent and isolated paths of the new age wellness industry, any system that does not look at all of the most fundamental variables is not likely to succeed.

The Medellin Wellness Protocol is an approach that integrates all of the most fundamental factors into a holistic system, and this is exactly what is required to achieve positive results in the shortest possible time.

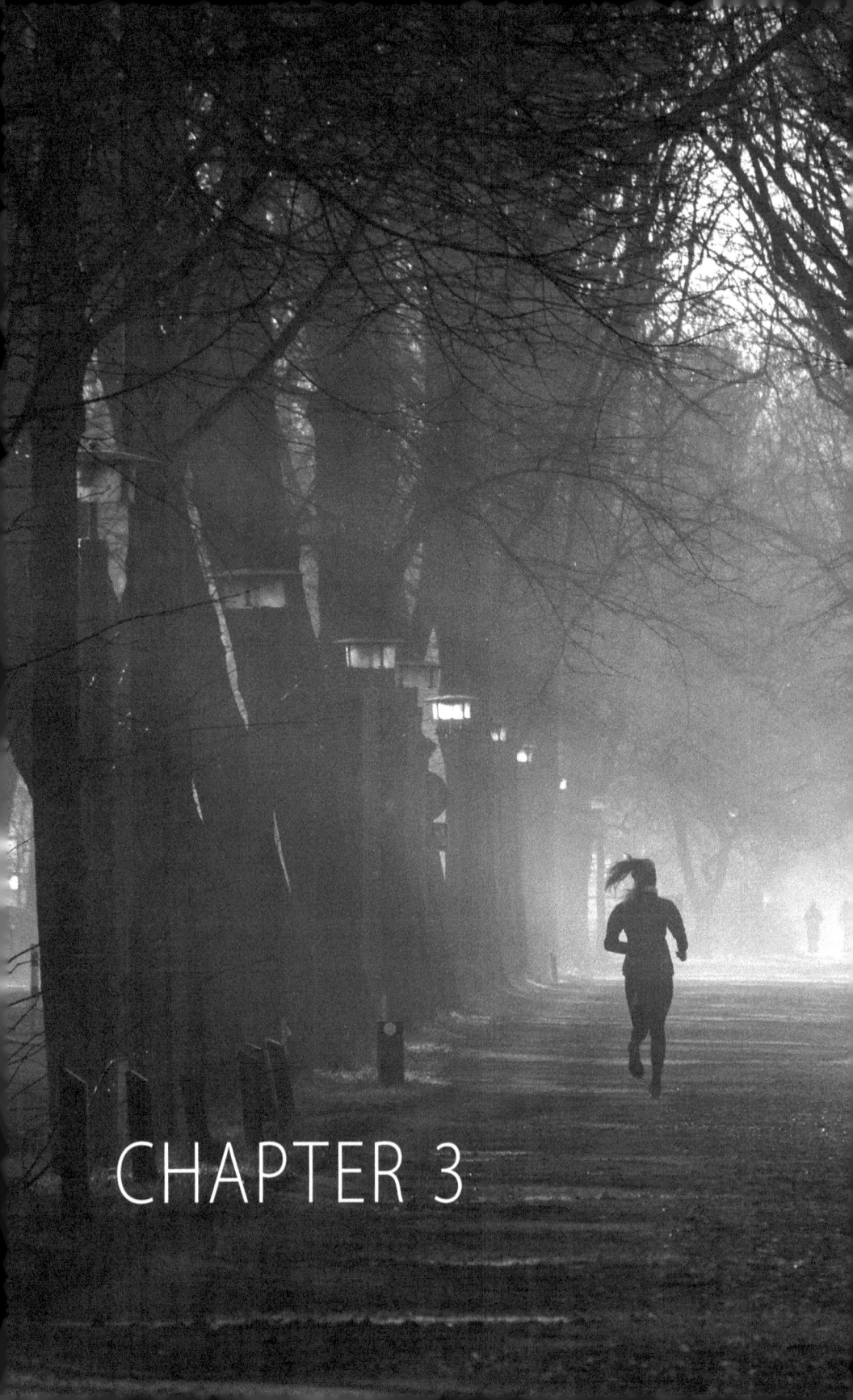

CHAPTER 3

Feedback Cycles

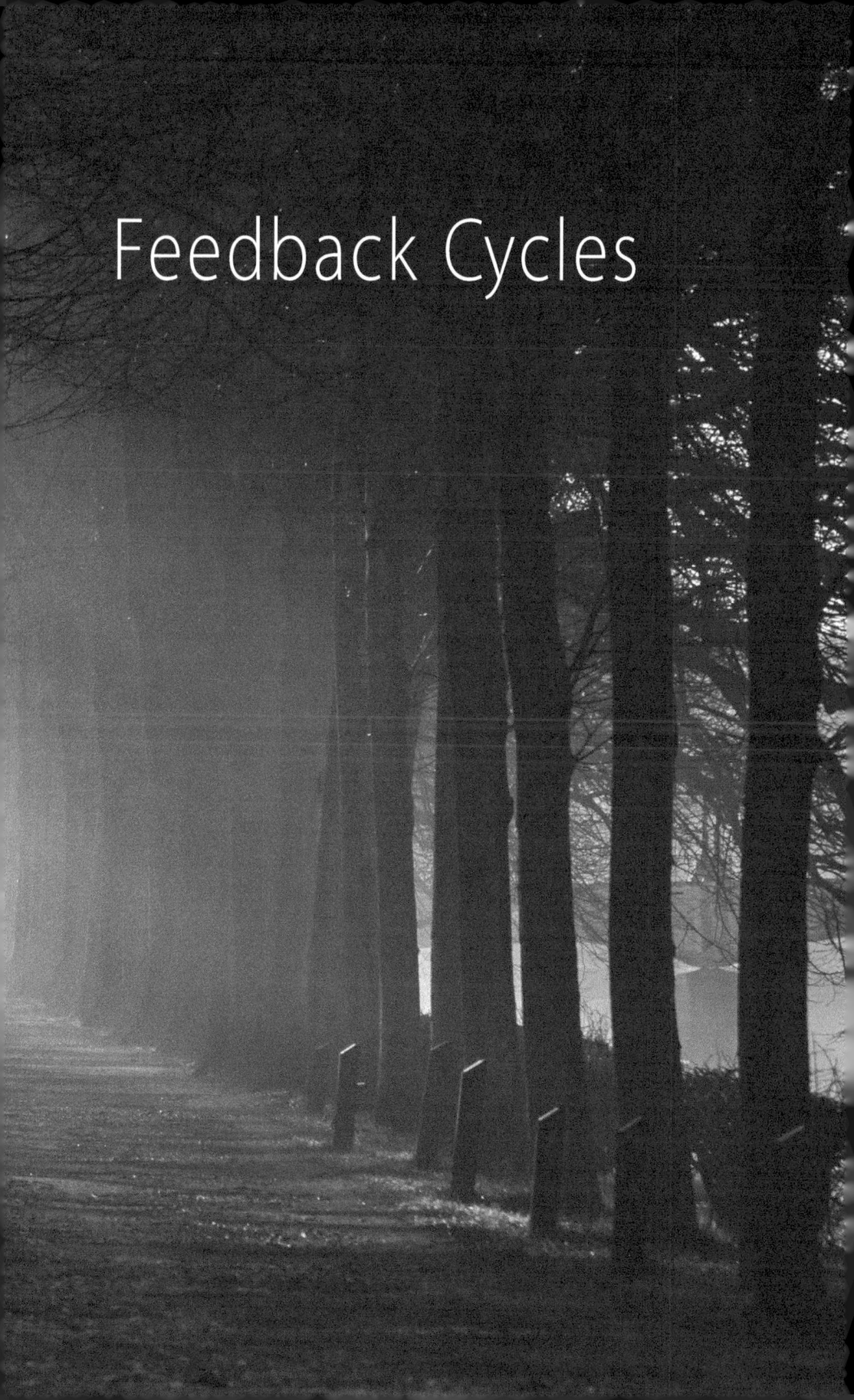

There exists in nature a powerful mechanism known as feedback cycles which can be applied in a much broader sense to our overall health and wellness. Feedback cycles are powerful biofeedback loops that create momentum which then serves to increase and reinforce each variable so that the original direction is amplified.

We can create our own feedback cycles and the Five Fundamental Factors of the Medellin Wellness Protocol are designed specifically to initiate what can be described as the 'positive feedback cycle'.

In other words, each factor of the program supports and promotes the other elements and each element strengthens the others, creating a powerful positive feedback loop. So, the maximum effect is achieved by applying all elements so that they can work in concert.

Feedback cycles and how they operate offer a very important understanding for us on the path of wellness. Feedback cycles however can work in either a positive or negative direction. Most of us are all too familiar with the negative side of the feedback cycle which goes something like this.

One day we eat junk food and as a result we physically feel lousy and don't feel like exercising. As a result of not exercising and eating unhealthy food we feel more lousy, perhaps even depressed so we open the refrigerator for a 'temporary fix' to feel better. As we feel down and a bit depressed we do not feel motivated to exercise or read but instead to again return to that one thing that often helps us temporarily to feel better, which of course is one of the emotional foods like ice cream or potato chips.

Needless to say, this loop feeds itself and the result is the perpetuation of this cycle because after eating more crappy food we simply feel worse and then are less likely to exercise and then feel even more down and depressed. Does this sound familiar? It is extremely common to get on this negative feedback cycle until the only word to describe your state of mind is 'hopeless'.

But even if we are on this cycle now and feel really out of balance in life that the situation is far from hopeless. The reason lies in the other side of the feedback cycle spectrum that we discussed earlier called the Positive Feedback Cycle.

The Positive Feedback Cycle is the engine that drives transformation. It is the exact opposite of the Negative Feedback Cycle and serves to strengthen and reinforce your trajectory rather than weaken you. Let us take a look at the positive side of the feedback cycle.

One day we exercise and we feel great. This great feeling that we have after exercise motivates us to eat a piece of fruit instead of the normal doughnut we may have chosen. As a result of eating the fruit and exercising we feel mentally and physically energized and well. As we feel good mentally and physically we are motivated to exercise the next day which leads us to eat well which leads us to feel even better and improves our performance.

So, what do we need to know in order to make the feedback cycles work for us in a positive direction? Start with exercise!

For the Positive Feedback Cycle to activate, we simply start with exercise. Exercise is the most effective place to get on board the feedback train because exercise immediately makes us feel better and more optimistic. After a good workout

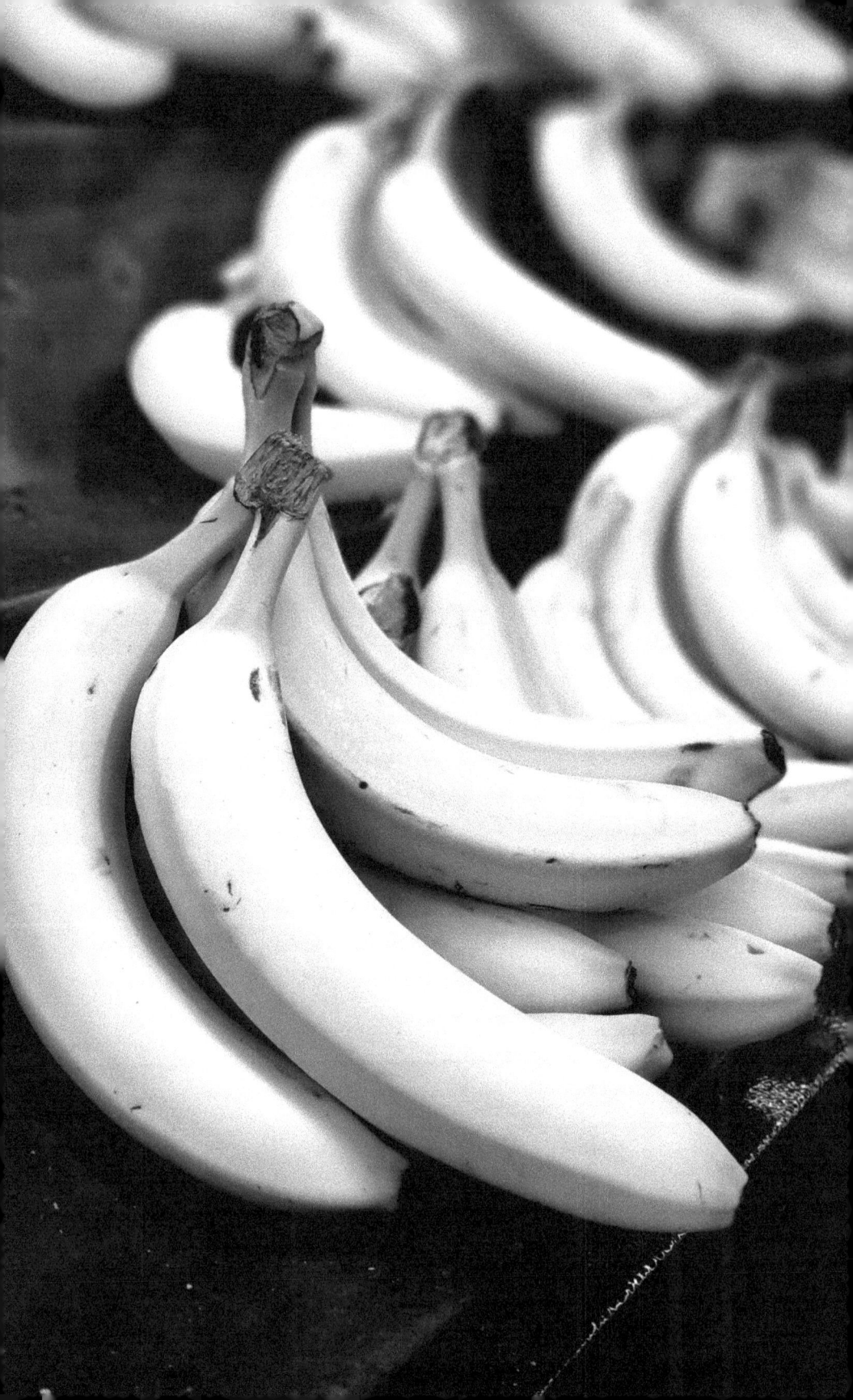

we are experiencing the benefits of good blood flow which invigorates us both physically and mentally while stimulating production of endorphins and helping us to detoxify.

Because exercise inevitably makes us feel better, it is unlikely that we will crave a candy bar as a post-workout snack. Instead, appreciating our new physical fitness, it seems natural and almost easy to eat smarter by choosing a banana or an apple instead. That decision to eat something more intelligent and healthy may seem trivial but in fact is extremely important because that step kicks the train into motion. Eating fruit and exercising starts the positive feeling of wellness and peace in the mind. Feeling great mentally the next day, the first thing we want to do is get to the gym or the pool or our yoga class. And the cycle continues carrying you to your destination of wellness.

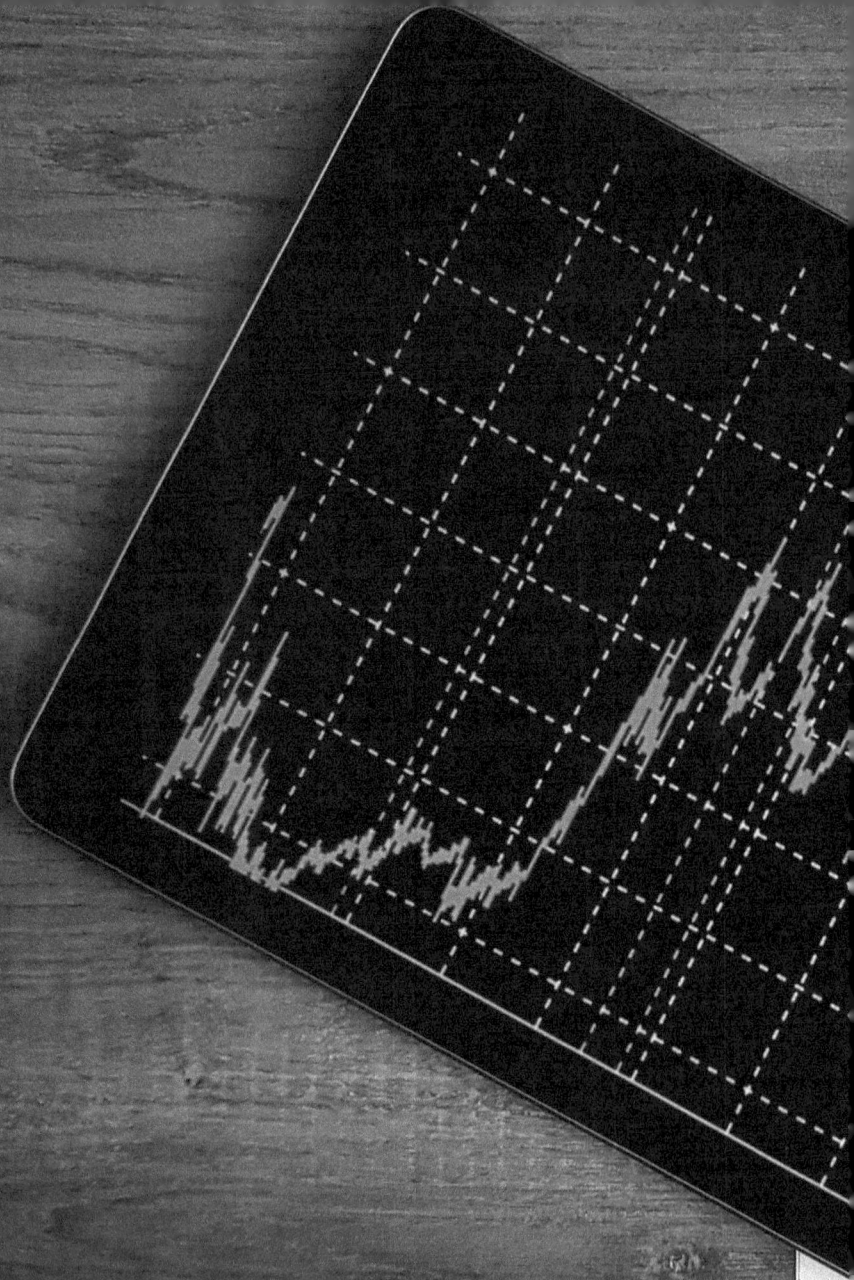

CHAPTER 4

The Big Corporate Obstacles to Wellness

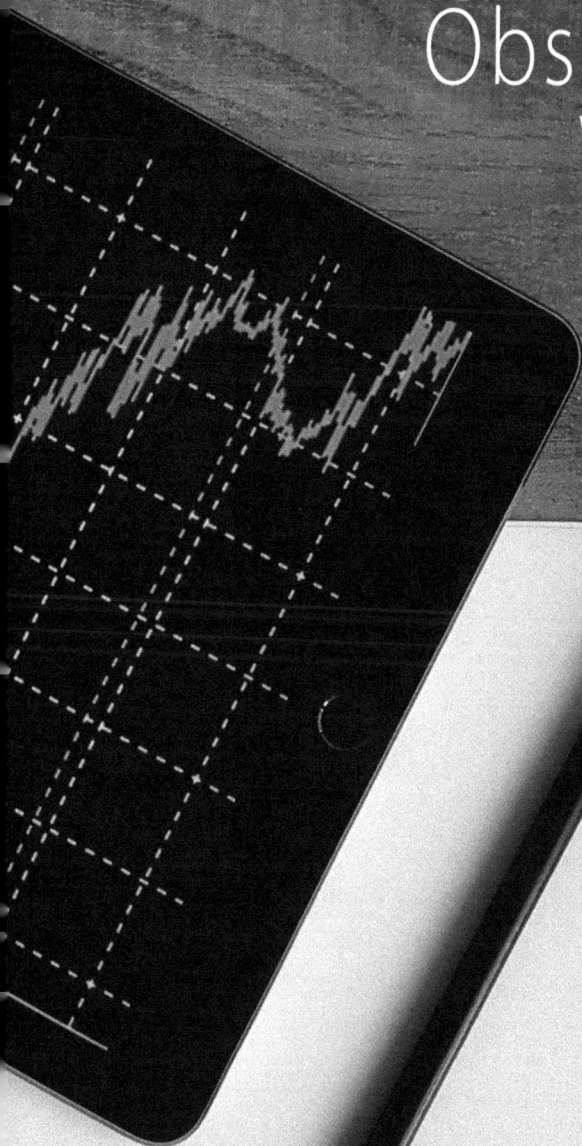

Our western society is driven economically by the idea of corporate profit. While there is nothing inherently wrong with profit, extreme greed and focus on profits over other factors can lead to perverse results. More importantly it creates obstacles to delivery to the masses of the simple truths that lead to health and wellness.

The first obstacle to be aware of is that we have corporate food giants promoting 'food' that is the most profitable for them regardless of the cost to society.

Companies that make money by selling foods that make people sick is a simple example of this. This consists of things that can be made from cheaply made, high profit, highly addictive ingredients such as corn syrup and white flour. Additionally, big corporations own massive operations such as dairy and cattle farms which produce dairy and meat products which are not beneficial to human health but which offer great profit potential, often due to misguided government subsidy.

The unspoken collusion between corporations and governments runs deep. The USDA, for example, is a government agency that is mandated to help protect and promote corporate agriculture interests and their 'food' products even though they are harmful for humans to consume. Driven by corporate interests and profit over everything the food corporations are driving the masses towards disease.

And we are all being told what to do and how to eat on TV, radio and online ads that are relentlessly playing to our emotional weaknesses. The result of the massive public relations and media campaigns financed by the giant corporations to promote unhealthy eating is predictable and demonstrated by the epidemic of obesity and cancer, as well as many other lifestyle driven health conditions.

Now here is the interesting part. As a result of eating these products people often become obese and develop a myriad of health problems such as cardiovascular disease and diabetes.

This is where big corporate pharma steps in with pills to treat everything.

Sure, the patient is told to diet and exercise in passing, but the primary focus of a doctor's visit for unhealthy people is never on the cause of the disease. That is because the pill approach is much more profitable and does not require a rethinking of the entire paradigm of how we live.

There is also no corporate profit to be made in the holistic approach of applying the factors for healthy living. Telling people to eat more fruit does not make anybody money because fruit is heavy and expensive to move and must be sold fresh, all factors that make them unprofitable for most corporations.

When there is a conflict of interest between making money and people's health we see almost always that making money wins and people's health is not considered.

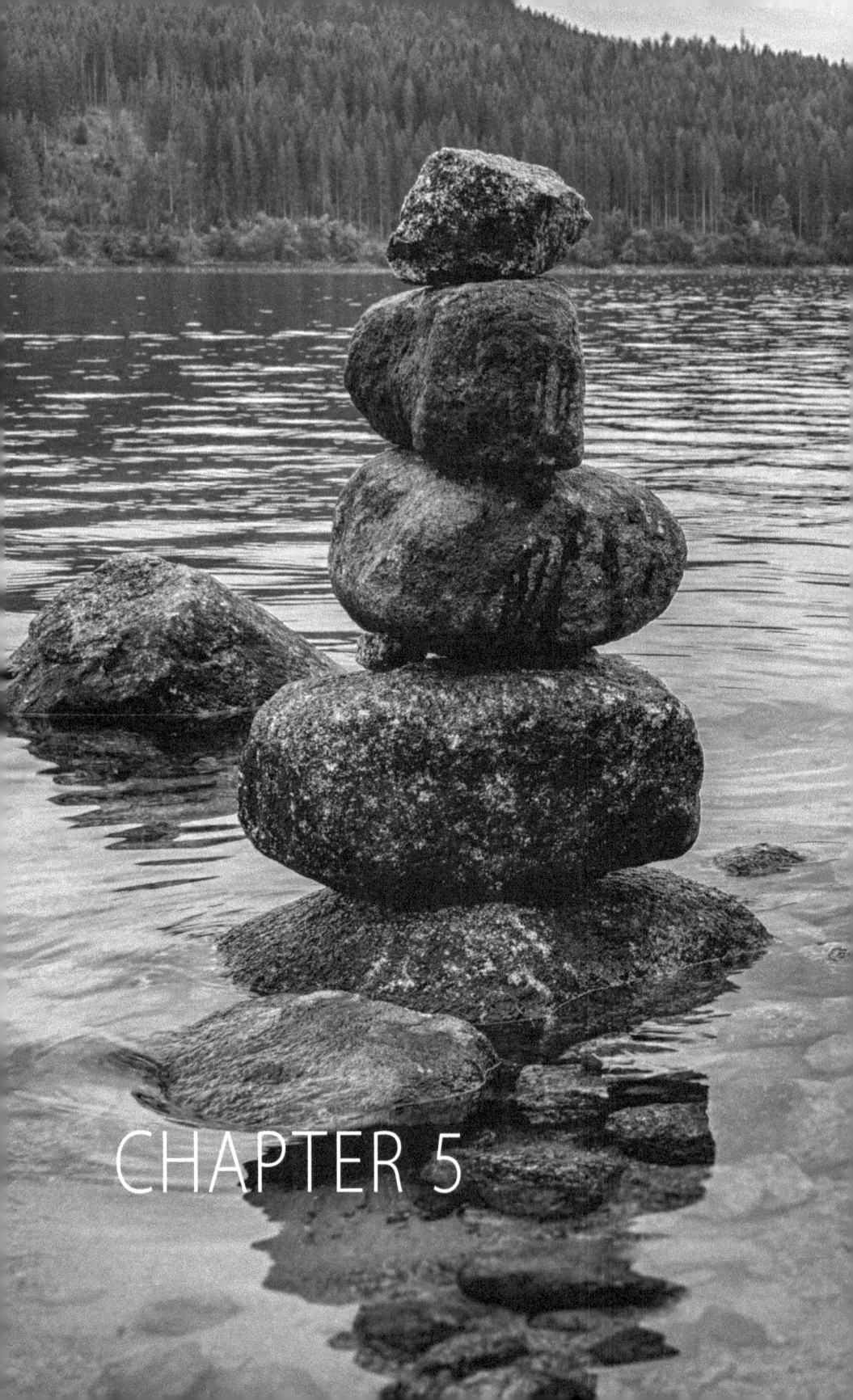

CHAPTER 5

The Five
Fundamental
Factors

So far this book has discussed and emphasized the importance of understanding feedback cycles. The reader has learned about the nature of feedback cycles and how they operate, with each variable responsible for reinforcing and strengthening each other variable and also the overall system. Now it is time to explore in specific detail the area called The Five Fundamental Factors of the Medellin Protocol which form the variables in the positive feedback cycle that we are looking to activate.

Each of these Fundamental Factors are essential for strengthening the immune system. In fact each of these factors alone are able to substantially act on the immune system in their own right. When put together these factors are responsible for helping a person activate the most powerful forces of healing and resilience possible.

FACTOR 1 – EXERCISE

Exercise starts us off on the positive feedback train and makes it all possible. Physical exertion profoundly improves the way our body works and this includes the functioning of the brain. The brain operates well only when inside a body that exercises. Exercise helps begin the feedback loop strengthening the body and the immune system while also providing endorphins and other factors that bring a sense of joy and positivity to life, which is the key to transformation.

Asking someone to first change their diet may initially often meet psychological and cultural resistance. In comparison, asking someone to begin to exercise often meets less resistance and so exercise is the best vector into the feedback loop. Exercise is best when enjoyable so that it becomes a joyful part of a person's day.

The body that is strong from exercise will find the expression of that strength as willpower. This willpower derived from exercise, along with the positive feeling mentioned earlier, are the drivers that improve every dimension of our life. Incorporating a daily exercise plan which will serve as the foundation for healthy and happy living is the first step.

FACTOR 2 – FOOD AND WATER INTAKE

'You are what you eat' is a common cliché but contains much truth. Our bodies, including our brains, are formed by what we consume and function for better or worse depending on the materials provided. There is much accuracy in the metaphor that food is the fuel to the human body and just as an engine will break down with poor quality or contaminated gasoline so will the body break down with poor quality and contaminated food. There is a reason why the airlines do not put diesel fuel into their jet engines which is of course that the engines would be damaged or destroyed.

It is impossible to overstate the importance of eating according to biology and anatomy. As will be discussed in detail, human beings are primates and have a certain digestive system designed to eat a very specific diet. Just like any other animal in nature is sickened when given an unnatural diet, so too are humans when they feed themselves in a way that is not aligned to our anatomy and physiology.
When the factor of exercise is reinforced by the factor of food selection, the positive feedback cycle begins to really get moving. These two factors alone work together in a way that provides truly significant results. When the other factors are added into the equation things really get powerful.

FACTOR 3 – THE MIND: ATTITUDE AND AWARENESS

The mind is directly connected to the immune system. The field of psychoneuroimmunology has been around for decades, demonstrating the direct link between a person's state of consciousness or mood and the functioning of the immune system. Thus it is entirely accurate to say that every single thought a person has either poisons them or heals them.

While it is true that *'we are what we eat'* it is also true that *'we are what we think.'* How a person uses their mind, or allows their mind to use them, will determine a person's reality and perception of life.

Unlike what most people believe, that external events determine internal state of mind, i.e. people get wet when it rains, the real fact is that the mind itself determines the state of consciousness independent of external events. This is why one person feels down and depressed when it rains and a different person feels happy as they consider how the region needed rain and how it may help the local animals drink water.

People who live out their life as one unconscious pattern after another and get sad when it rains just because that is what people say should happen, are not as powerful as they could be and this weakness leads to more belief that the external world is responsible. In comparison when a person who, through meditation, gains access to the programming levels of their mind, they can literally transform their present moment and their future.

It is not an overstatement to suggest that every single thought we think has a profound physical and mental effect. As we learn how to achieve greater awareness over our minds we can begin to dissolve patterns of negativity and replace them with harmonizing and healing visualizations.

When the factors of exercise and diet are reinforced with a well-programmed and focussed mind, the positive feedback cycle really accelerates.

FACTOR 4 – REST

As people struggle to make ends meet in this challenging environment, one of the first things to be sacrificed is sleep. Many people simply must work too hard, often more than one job, just to support their family and sleep becomes a luxury that they literally cannot afford. This is highly unfortunate because sleep and rest are not optional and if sacrificed will force the person to pay a heavy price eventually. Sleep is where all healing and nervous energy restoration take place. Sleep deprivation, as will be discussed, has very negative effects on the immune system and overall health.

As much as the body needs exercise the body also needs rest. For those who have trouble sleeping it is good to learn that exercise, intelligent diet and mental awareness are all very helpful to achieve deep and restorative sleep. A body that does not exercise will not be tired enough to want to sleep as there will be too much nervous system energy that has been unreleased, which translates into an active mind.

Sleep is not something a person should *try* to achieve. Instead a person should simply enjoy the relatively relaxing and comfortable environment of their bed and allow themselves to *fall into* sleep without any effort or struggle.

When the factors of exercise, diet, and mind are reinforced by good rest, the energy systems of the body are all directed to the feedback loop which then gains even more momentum.

FACTOR 5 – LIVING ORGANICALLY AND THE ENVIRONMENTAL FACTORS

Factors like air quality and exposure to environmental and personal care poisons can make a big difference to our ability to live and age with good health. Many things in life are not realized to be poisons because they are so commonly used. However it is time now to recalibrate that perception and understand the science and chemistry of poisoning the body.

It is important to be aware that many products that are part of our everyday lives that are not perceived as toxic are, in fact, toxic. As we will discuss in more detail later, all perfumes, cleaning sprays, shampoos, artificial foods, baby powders and such are toxic compounds that enter into our human system and cause damage because they are not natural to the human body.

We absorb environmental pollution and toxins through our five sense organs which then transport the damaging materials or energy waves into our physical body. Once in our physical body these toxins can cause things like inflammation, immune response, a variety of negative effects and eventually health conditions.

THE BODY INGESTS TOXINS IN THE FOLLOWING WAYS:

Inhalation – People are exposed to poisons and toxins which enter our bodies through the nose and lungs with noxious

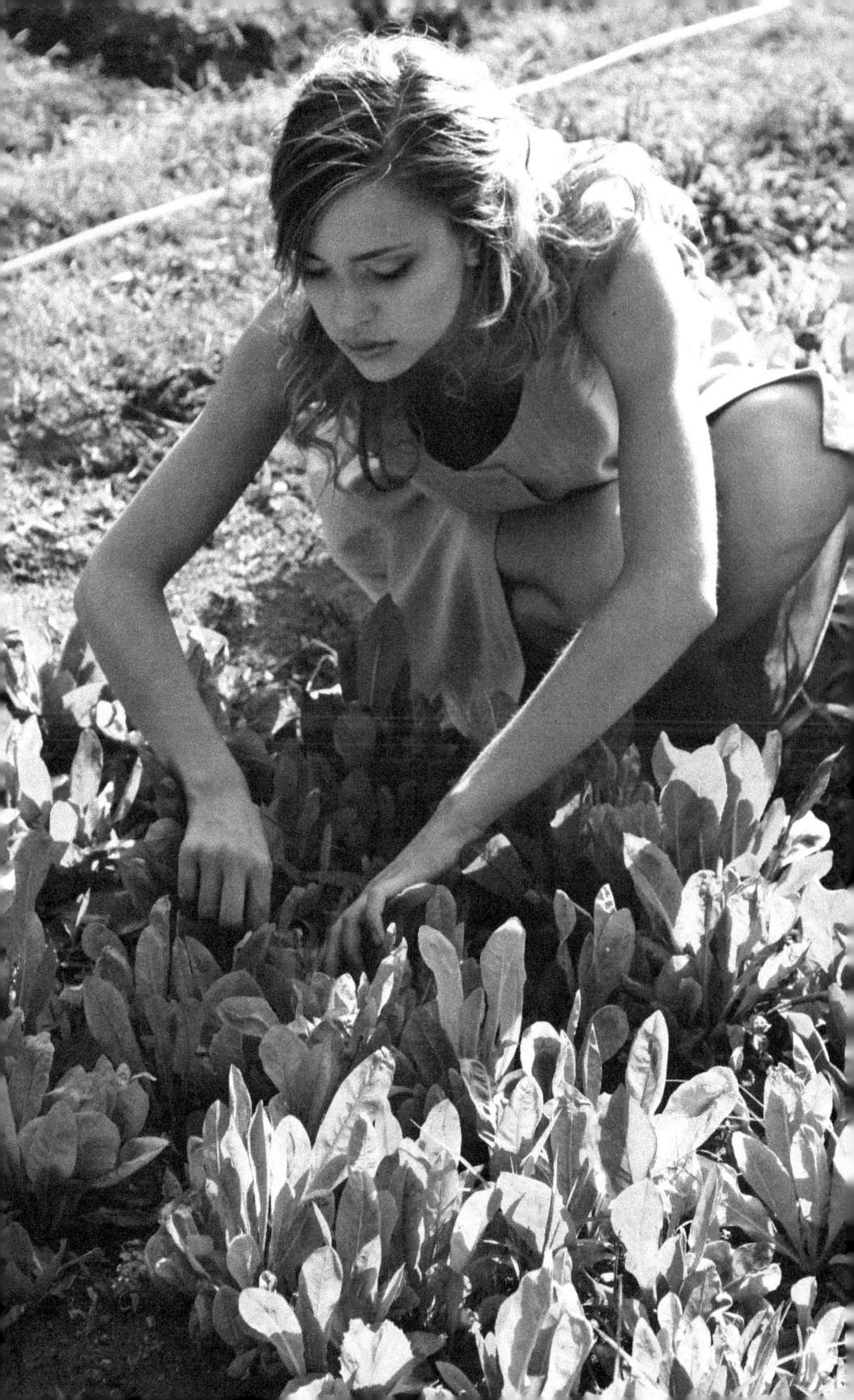

smells and chemicals of all varieties. Oftentimes the very odors that are perceived to be pleasant are the most dangerous such as perfumes and cleaning products with artificial scents.

Ingestion – The mouth is the primary organ of ingestion of matter and today is used to ingest many chemical compounds that are unnatural. The body sees things only as 'food' or 'poison' and many different things that masquerade as foods are actually poisons as far as the body is concerned. Many products that are disguised as good are simply means for poisons to infiltrate the body and wreak havoc.

The Skin – The skin is a *sponge* that literally absorbs whatever it is exposed to. Skin products and perfumes as well as all kinds of creams and lotions are used by the masses and unfortunately very little attention is paid to what is actually in them. A person should consider putting something on our skin as similar to eating it because the skin absorbs whatever touches it directly into the bloodstream.

The Eyes – Exposure to negative energy through the eyes in the form of violence or emotionally charged movies disturbs our nervous system. While it may be impossible to limit exposure to popular culture completely, it is wise for a person to do their best to mitigate the amount of time spent exposed to violence or sensational news on the TV or computer screens. Exposure to beauty and nature should be encouraged as much as possible.

The Ears – Like the eyes, the ears are very susceptible to absorbing negative waves that disrupt health and balance. Certain music and TV programs subject the ears and subconscious minds to a barrage of negative waves that are best avoided.

When all of these Five Fundamental Factors are aligned a person will begin to experience an ever stronger and more powerful momentum behind them almost as if there is a wind filling their sails. As these factors continue to reinforce themselves they also grow ever deeper roots into a person's good habits and subconscious mind and these roots soon grow so strong that they are never uprooted regardless of the external pull leveraged on them.

CHAPTER 6

Why this Approach?

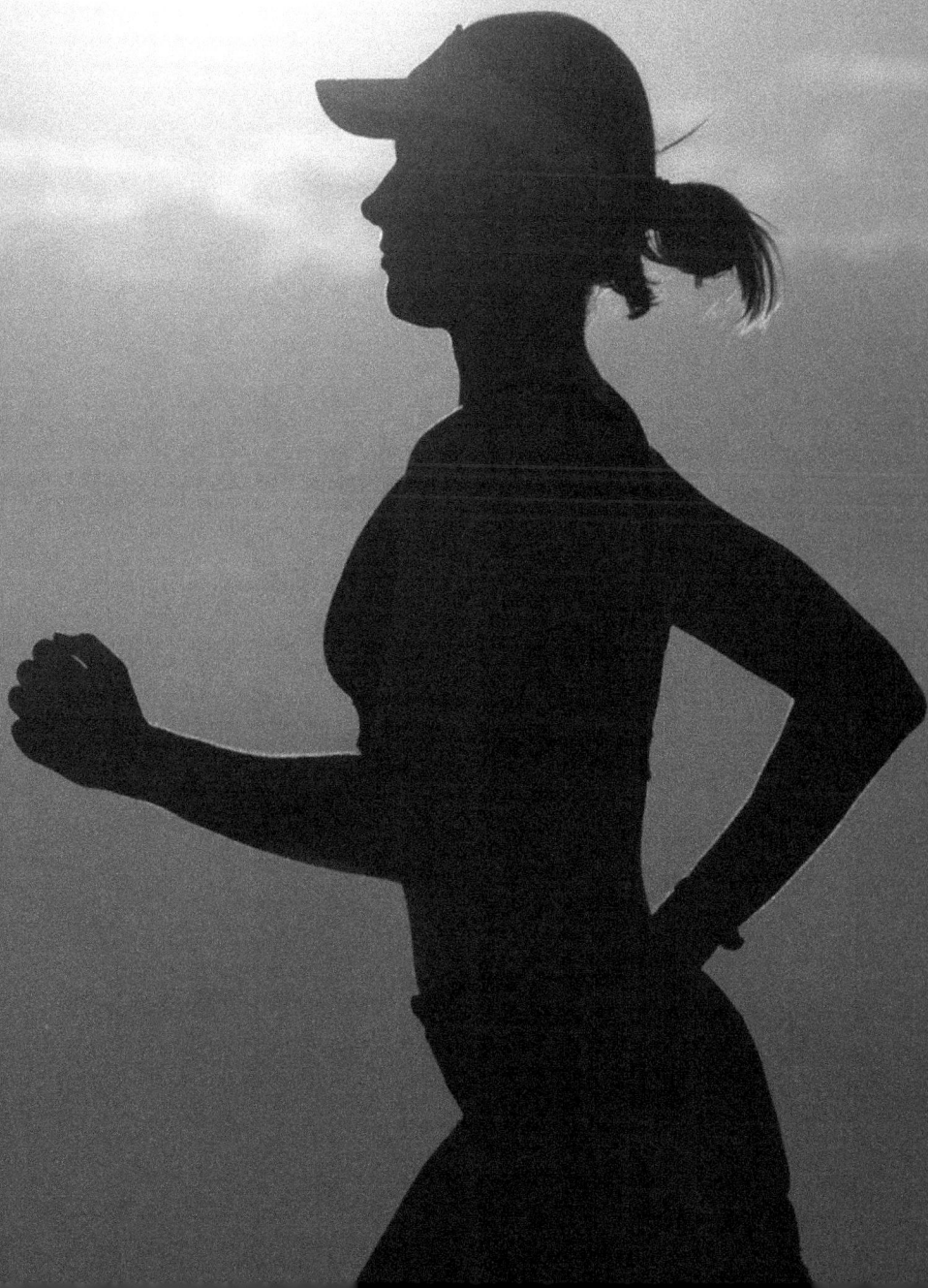

This book represents what some might call an alternative way of approaching health challenges that is quite different from the mainstream western allopathic approach (i.e. treatment of the problem with drugs) as we shall see.

Allopathy looks at symptoms as the primary problem and believes that when symptoms are eliminated that the problem has been resolved. For example upon going to a medical doctor for a complaint of a headache the doctor will reflexively prescribe you some pharmaceutical and if your headache goes away will consider the case resolved.

In other words the paradigm is suggesting or even dictating that the cause of your headache or shoulder pain is a deficiency of Ibuprofen or OxyContin.

This view is not valid because #1 the human body is healthy when it is free from the need to take drugs. No chemical that makes a healthy person sick can make a sick person healthy. And #2 symptoms are not the disease but rather an expression of an underlying cause. Because the cause is not being addressed and instead poisonous pharmaceuticals are administered, the true cause is suppressed and often results in much more serious conditions later on.

Unlike the western medical approach that dominates our culture and thinking about disease, the Medellin Wellness Protocol is multidimensional and completely interested in cause as opposed to just symptoms. When cause is addressed the symptoms dissipate.

According to the viewpoint of the Medellin Wellness Protocol, the causes of most of mankind's most pervasive and degenerative conditions stem from a combination of lifestyle errors that must be addressed in concert.

We as a population are eating very far from our anatomical design while at the same time living sedentary lifestyles. Add to that sleep deprivation and exposure to toxins in our food and immediate environment, and we now have the perfect storm.

The ability to see the cause of this epidemic of degeneration and disease is essential to our ability to heal ourselves or help others to heal. The Medellin Wellness Protocol is designed to address the many possible causes of disease symptoms so that the body can return to its natural state which is health.

Put simply The Medellin Protocol will teach you the five components, known as the Five Fundamental Factors that address cause and create the feedback mechanisms that are so important to reversing disease processes, regaining full health and preventing disease.

CHAPTER 7

The Upside and Downside of Allopathy

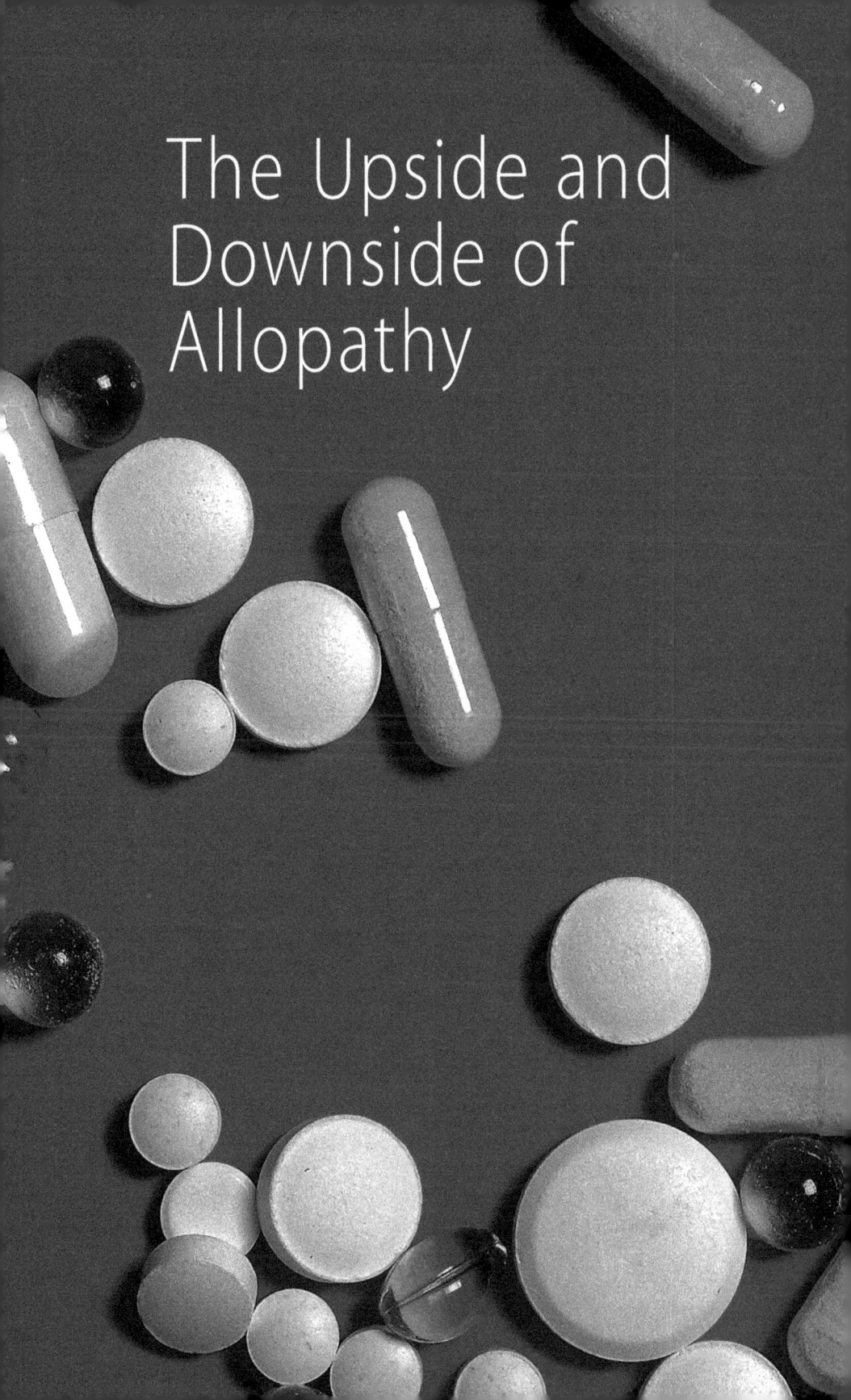

In the following chapter much of the approach taken by allopathy will be criticised. However before we get into what could be considered the glaring weakness of this system of treatment, it is important that we give credit where credit is due. It is necessary first and foremost to acknowledge the aspects of modern allopathic medicine that have indeed provided a huge benefit to humanity.

Trauma care, emergency rooms and surgery are the primary areas where modern medicine indeed is a marvel and a true wonder. One would want without question to be under the supervision and care of allopathic medicine in situations of life or death. When we are injured severely with a car accident or a bullet wound or any life threatening injury, there is no better place to be than a well-funded western allopathic medical hospital.

Emergency department physicians perform incredible work every day with their capacity to stabilize and perform life-saving procedures. All must have a profound respect for the skillful physicians saving lives every day.

Another area where physicians are essential is with performing necessary surgical procedures to repair traumatic injuries such as fractures. Although surgeons perform many unnecessary surgeries it is clearly true that surgical treatment is often necessary and life-saving.

Having sung the praises of the valuable aspects of modern medicine it is time to address the weaknesses that are creating epidemics of health crises in our society.

In fact let it be known first off that dealing with medical professionals requires extreme caution, rather than blind obedience. Dr. Robert Mendelsohn, former Dean of Tufts

University Medical School, states in his work, *Confessions of a Medical Heretic*, 'Hospitals are like war zones; they are to be avoided at all cost.'

Dr. Mendelsohn also observes in his book that this system has strived for and attained an almost church-like status in our culture. Medical doctors, he maintains, are considered the unquestioned experts in wellbeing and often their advice is taken as gospel and never challenged.

Doctors often have very little patience for questions for a few reasons. One primary reason is that doctors in hospitals and clinics are completely overbooked and, in a hurry to see the next patient.

Another reason a doctor does not like questions from patients is that simply put they may not have a precise answer to what is causing your problem. Much of medicine is educated guesswork. Thus, you might hear that the cause is either a 'virus' or something labeled as 'autoimmune' and this is convenient because it is medical sounding enough for us to not question although it says nothing about the cause of our condition.

And then to make it worse, after not addressing the cause the western medical approach is always the same: treat you with drugs and see what happens.

Instead of addressing the cause of a person's medical symptoms the allopathic physician instead decides to attack the symptom with a pharmaceutical. The fallacy is the idea that we can help a person to heal by introducing poisonous chemicals that we know very little about into their system, and in many cases, not knowing if the medication being prescribed is appropriate since the diagnosis may not be correct.

So why is this approach so popular? Simply put the western approach is more convenient! The western approach is a much easier answer for most patients as well as doctors. For example, if you have what they call gastroesophageal reflux disease (heartburn from acid backing up from your stomach) it is much easier to say 'take this pill' than to explain to the patient that 'the food you are eating is garbage, you are eating three times as much of it as you should and you are grossly overweight so you don't need a pill, you need to completely change your lifestyle!'

Even if the doctor is aware of all this, from the doctor's perspective, they believe that most patients don't want to hear that. They also believe that people probably won't comply anyway so the pill makes more sense. However the big problem here is that the pills themselves are foreign chemicals to the body that have predictably harmful effects. This is the ultimate flaw of modern medicine.

As argued by Dr. Robert Mendelsohn in his book *Confessions of a Medical Heretic*, the allopathic medical community is responsible for much more sickness and death than we might suspect.

Voltaire in the 1700s put it very succinctly when he said 'Doctors put drugs of which they know little into bodies of which they know less to treat diseases of which they know nothing'. And Voltaire said this: 'The art of **medicine** consists in amusing the patient while nature cures the disease'. It is fascinating to reflect on how true both of those statements are today.

This is true because when Voltaire says Nature he is referring to the body's own self-healing capacities which are self-evident.

On a superficial level think about the fact that if you cut your finger your body has the capacity to heal itself and it will always heal of its own accord without outside interference. What happens superficially also happens at the deeper levels.

Let us look at another example that may help illustrate our point relating to high blood pressure- or cholesterol-lowering drugs. These drugs do not address the causes of the underlying condition (i.e. poor diet and lack of exercise) and patients are told to take the prescriptions for the remainder of their life. The physician who prescribes these drugs is essentially declaring that a person will be sick forever and that drugs will be required for their entire life.

Again, taking a pill may be a much more convenient approach than suggesting changes in what a person should eat or how to live, but they do not make a person healthier – rather they create complications in their own right.

To be fair, it is certainly possible to have high blood pressure or cardiovascular disease with a healthy lifestyle – but it is very rare and these conditions are highly associated with poor diet and lack of exercise.

When was the last time your doctor suggested that you change your way of eating to resolve your health issue? Usually never, because in medical school they don't focus on the undeniable fact that there is a relationship between diet and health. This denial of dietary influence on health is another one of the major weaknesses of the allopathic system.

Of course the problem is naturally about money and our system is one where doctors are paid more when there are more sick people in the world.

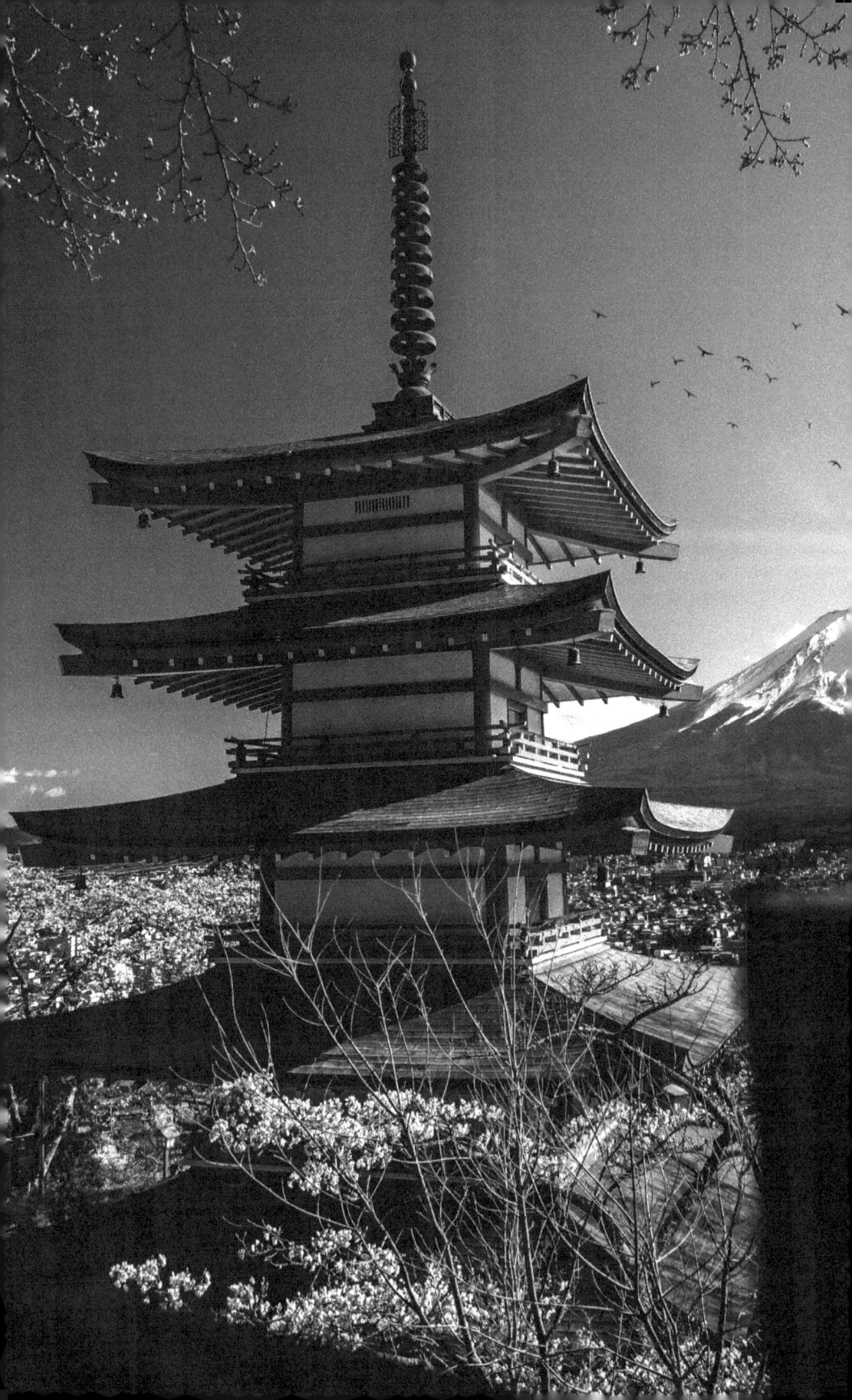

I once heard about an ancient Chinese medical system that was practiced in the old days. At that time in China the villagers would only pay their doctor on the years that they did *not* see them. In other words they paid their doctor for keeping them healthy. It was understood that if a person got sick and had to see the doctor that this means that the doctor did not do his job and thus did not deserve pay.

Imagine if insurance premiums were based on the degree to which you have a healthy lifestyle. The unfortunate reality is that medical doctors make more money when there are more sick people. Where is the incentive for them to help people get completely well? There is none. This is another problem with the western system and the results speak for themselves. Instead of helping people heal completely the allopathic system prefers to *manage* your symptoms with pharmaceuticals for your entire lifetime regardless of the many negative effects and the fact that the treatment provided is not by any means curative.

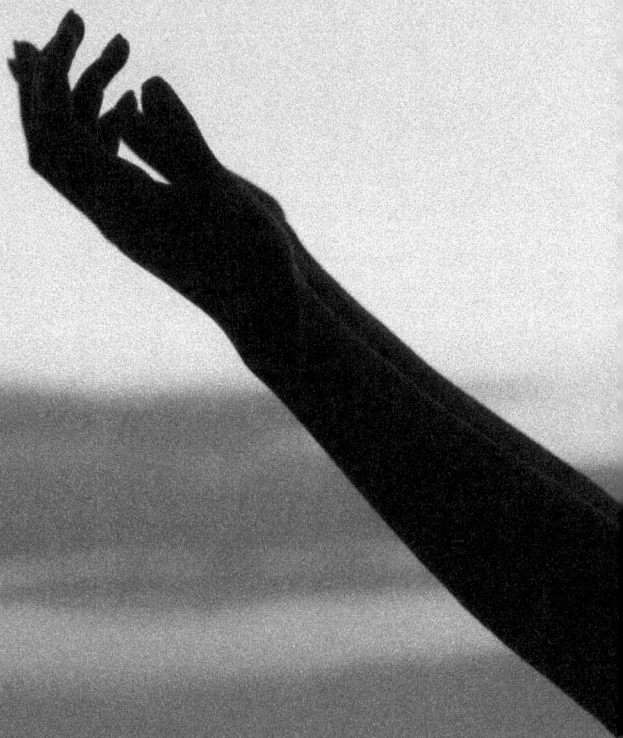

CHAPTER 8

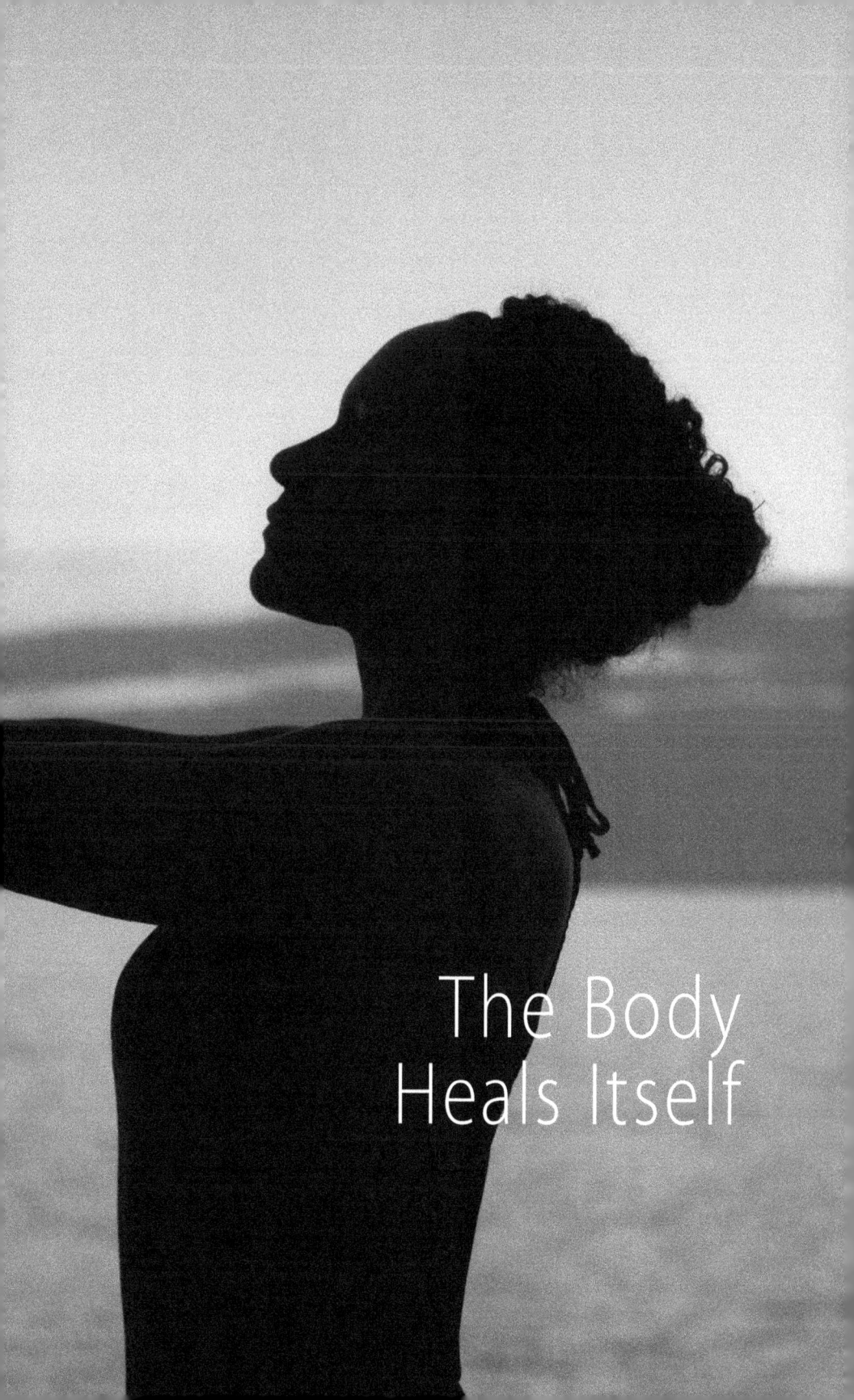

The Body
Heals Itself

One of the simplest and most profound facts about our body is that it is capable of healing itself. It is constantly engaged in the activities of healing and renewing our cells. We have been aware of this capacity since we were children when our cuts and scrapes would heal.

The body will heal itself always unless there is an obstacle to the healing process. In other words the body will heal itself unless we do something that interferes with the healing process. For example, if we scrape and bruise our leg in the exact same spot *every single day* then it will never heal. The body will not heal and symptoms will not be resolved if we continue to engage in actions that are causing the condition in the first place.

A smoker who has lung damage and continues to smoke is like a person with a bruised shin who continues to smash his shin every morning in the same place. And, a person with cardiovascular disease must stop eating greasy animal foods if they want to heal their vessels. Once we are able to stop the aggravating activities for at least a period of time the body usually begins immediately to affect healing and repair.

'As above so below' is a very important Chinese proverb that expresses the idea that whatever operations one can observe on the superficial dimensions are also operating the same way in the deeper dimensions. So, what we see happening with our skin and its ability to heal itself is also happening for our vessels and muscles and internal organs.

In order to stop aggravating the processes that are causing the health issue or symptoms we must align our body to biology, anatomy and chemistry.

We do this by applying the Five Fundamental Factors of the Medellin Wellness Protocol of how to eat, how to exercise and rest, how to use our mind, and how to live organically and protect our personal environment from unnecessary toxic exposure.

CHAPTER 9

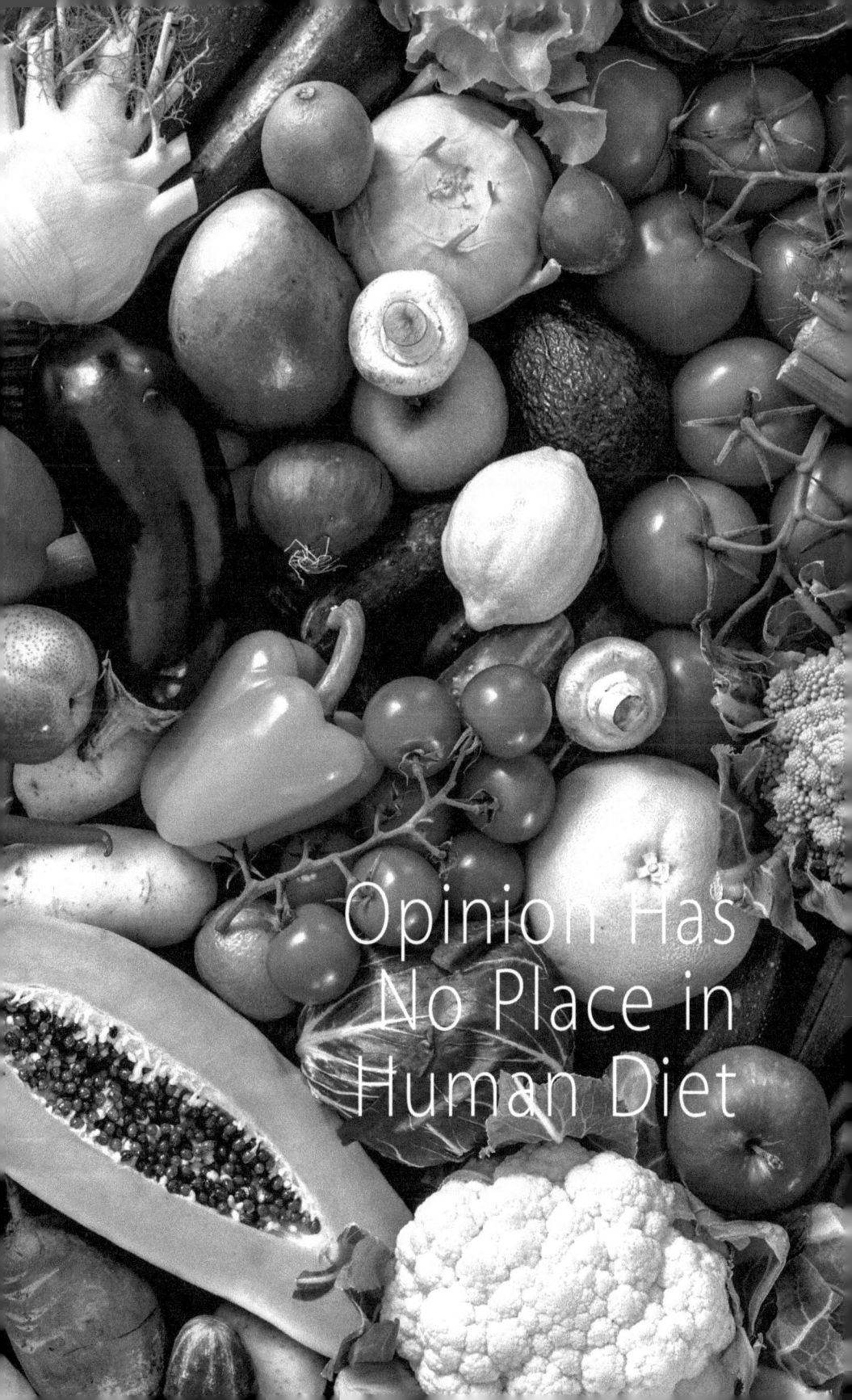

Opinion Has
No Place in
Human Diet

One of the most challenging aspects for people trying to determine the best dietary regimen is the fact that there are many different, conflicting and confusing opinions. What's worse is that these differing opinions come from people who are either medical doctors or highly trained academics designated to be experts in the field of nutrition. The subject of nutrition is a diverse set of opinions spread around in books, the media, and medical literature and as a result it is difficult to know what to listen to.

Everyone finds themselves in a situation where Dr. 'X' says one thing while Dr. 'Y' says something else while Dr. 'Z' has an entirely different opinion. With all of these experts with advanced degrees contradicting each other how is a person to distinguish between these opinions for levels of truth and determine what is actually the best? *How is it that the opinions are so conflicting?*

Of the many opinions regarding human diet and nutrition, one must be fact. The other opinions must be false because human beings like all animals in nature have one genetically and naturally designated perfect diet. This is fact without exception as shown in nature.

So many experts giving their wide spectrum of opinions on the human diet suggest the most *unscientific* of all possible content. Many experts and doctors are using scientific language to make highly unscientific statements.

Is it valid or responsible or even possible for me to have an opinion declaring something that is scientifically demonstrated to be wrong? Of course, the answer is no.

All opinions must be based on fact-based reality. For example, it would be absurd for someone to have an opinion that the speed of light is 10 miles an hour when the science demonstrates otherwise.

Now we can look at other scientifically observed facts like for example what do certain animals eat in nature? If we are a marine biologist and we study dolphins in their natural state for 20 years and observe that dolphins eat fish primarily then would it be valid for somebody who has no experience with dolphins to have an opinion about what dolphins eat? Say for example this person says, 'NO! My opinion is that dolphins only eat apples in nature!' That would be absurd. Nobody is allowed to have an 'opinion' about what dolphins eat because they eat what they are genetically and naturally designed for.

We can use this example for every single species on earth and demonstrate that for every single species on earth what they eat is observable and related to their anatomical structure.

What these animals eat is a scientific fact based on anatomy and physiology and of course observable in nature. This is as true for what humans as for tigers or antelopes or insects or dolphins.

As a species, humankind has the same digestive structure as other great apes and therefore it is a scientific truth that we are designed to eat as close to what they eat as our environment allows. We are basically fruit eaters by nature as we shall later discuss. But one thing is certain, which is that opinions about our diet based on any other method is not relevant to the question of what humans naturally eat.

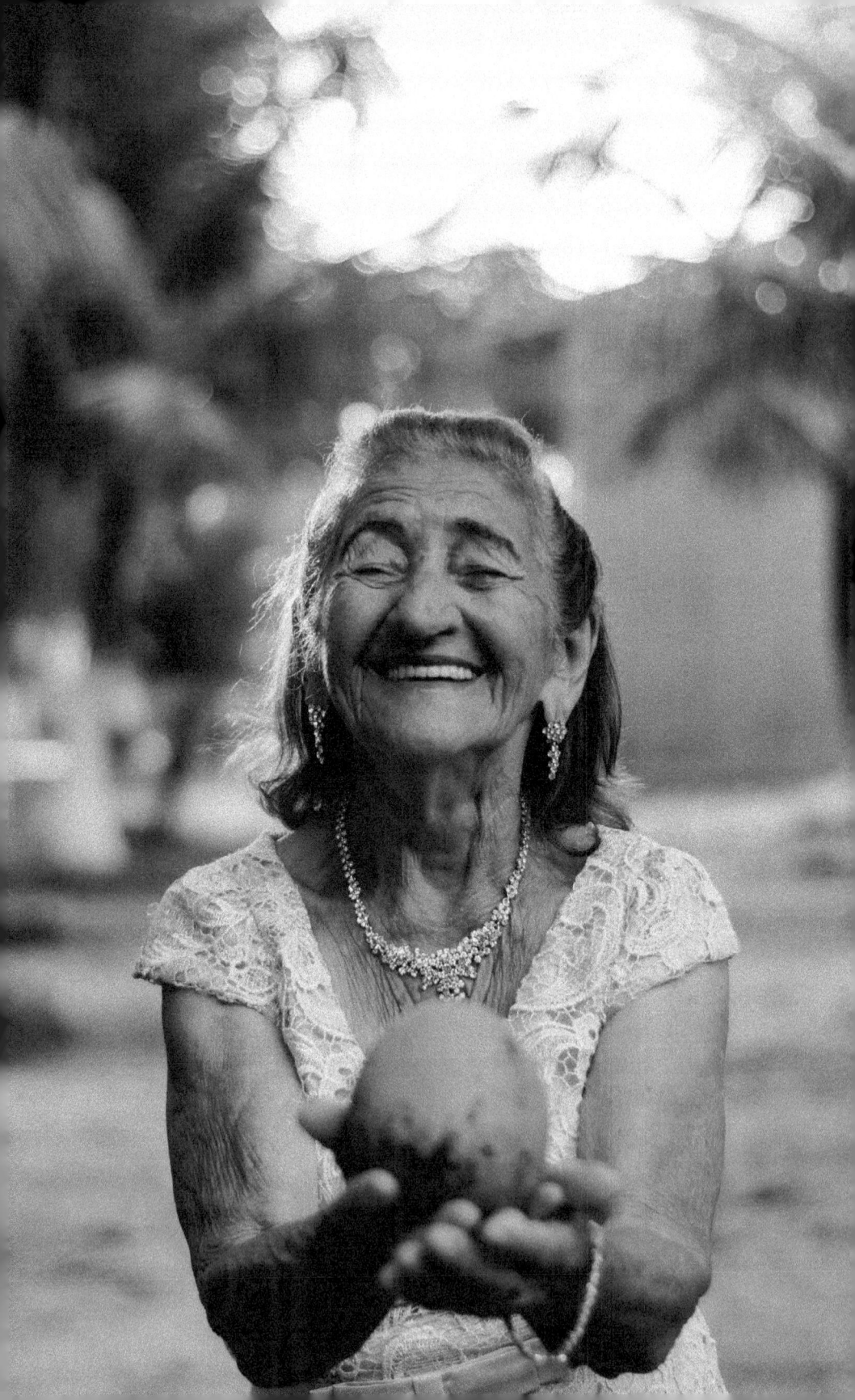

The author worked at a primate center in Miami and observed that the veterinarians were in charge of the diet of the great apes. The diet prescribed by the vets in order to keep the chimpanzees, gorilla, orangutans and gibbons in perfect health was 100% fruits. Not one time in the years that the author worked there was observed a great ape ever being given anything other than fruit. Never.

Why is that? Because it is well known that the best way to make an animal sick is to violate its biologically indicated dietary preferences and force the animal to eat something it is not designed to consume. The veterinarians (doctors) are in charge of the health of these animals and they are using the correct biological diet as the number one way to guarantee optimum health.

How is it then that we have applied this logic to great apes and animals in zoos but not to ourselves and our children? We do not seem too interested in the type of species we are and the diet of its anatomical design.

CHAPTER 10

Morris Charts

Line Chart

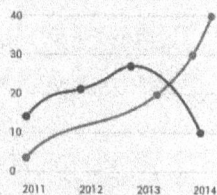

Area Chart

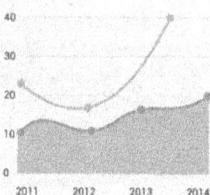

Bar Chart

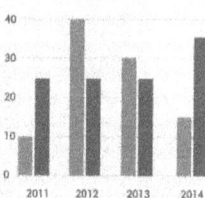

Donut

Sparkline Charts

Line Chart

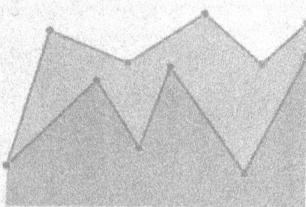

Bar Chart

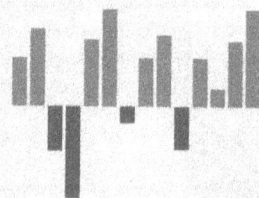

Pie Chart

Easy Pie Charts

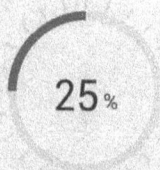

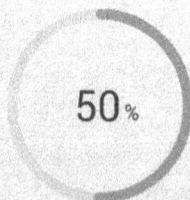

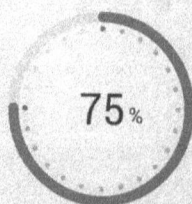

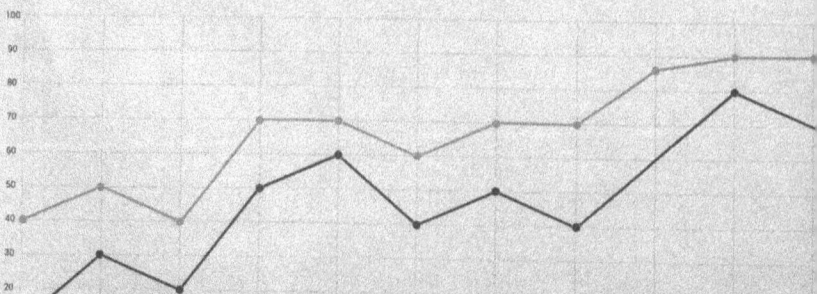

The Incomplete Focus of Nutrition in Wellness

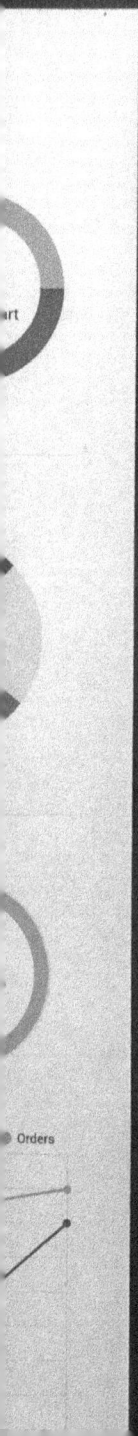

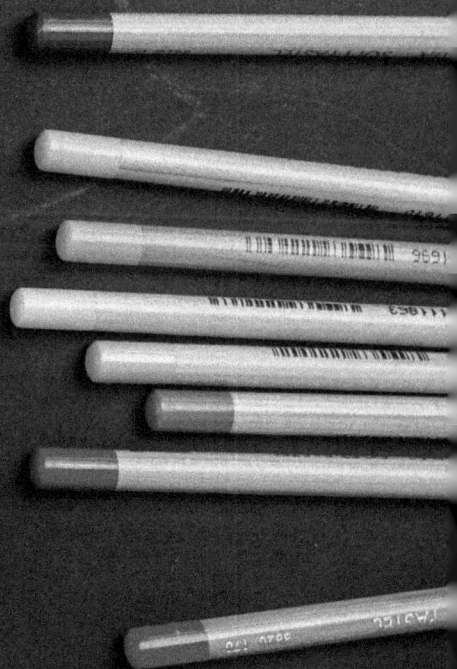

The subject of nutrition is based on the premise that getting enough nutritional elements is the key to dietary success. According to this way of thinking the most important thing is to make sure that every day you receive a certain amount of nutrition.

There is no question that we need enough calories to live. Certainly, calorie intake is a fundamental consideration because we need fuel. Nutrients on the other hand are not fuel and in fact play very different roles from that of directly powering the body. Vitamins are needed for enzymatic activity and minerals are required as electrolytes and for structural support, but these are not fuels. Amino acids are used to build protein and they also play important roles as neurotransmitters while fatty acids are needed for insulation of nerves as well as membranes of cells but none of these factors run the engine of the body.

Clearly nutrition is important and a lot of important things will not function well or at all if we do not get our spectrum of nutrients in a viable form. However it is incomplete to think of nutrition as simply the subject of getting enough nutritional factors.

The story is incomplete because most people are being damaged gravely by the food selections they are making and this damage is far and above worse than any small nutritional gain. In other words when we glean some nutrients from within an overall destructive food choice like animal foods we take one step forward and three steps back away from our destination of wellness and immune strength.

The Standard American Diet that has been exported around the world, and particularly to the UK, includes massive amounts of dead animal foods mixed with refined complex carbohydrates and very little fruits or vegetables where the nutrition is found. This is a highly damaging diet regardless of whether nutritional elements exist within these selections.

Typical food choices are actually injurious to the body in several major ways. So by relying on the idea that the primary thing to consider is nutritional elements we are missing the most important factor contributing to people's disease and symptoms which is direct damage from the food itself.

Ironically, even with the focus on nutrition, the vast majority of what people are eating has almost no nutrition whatsoever. This is, as the reader will soon learn, because nutritional elements can only be well integrated into the body from whole foods that have not been cooked which is to say, destroyed.

Studies have shown that the effect on your immune system by taking chemical vitamin C is nothing compared to eating fresh citrus. The complexity of nutrition cannot be reduced to a couple of handfuls of chemicals given letter names and then manufactured in a laboratory.

Fortified foods are not any better. When we eat something that has been artificially fortified with vitamins and minerals those elements are not readily absorbed by the body because they are not in the form of a whole food. The other problem with these fortified manufactured foods is that they have been refined to remove all of the valuable micronutrients that existed in the natural version of the food.

We want to get our nutrition from real natural fresh food. Period. But, the lack of nutrients in manufactured food is only part of the story.

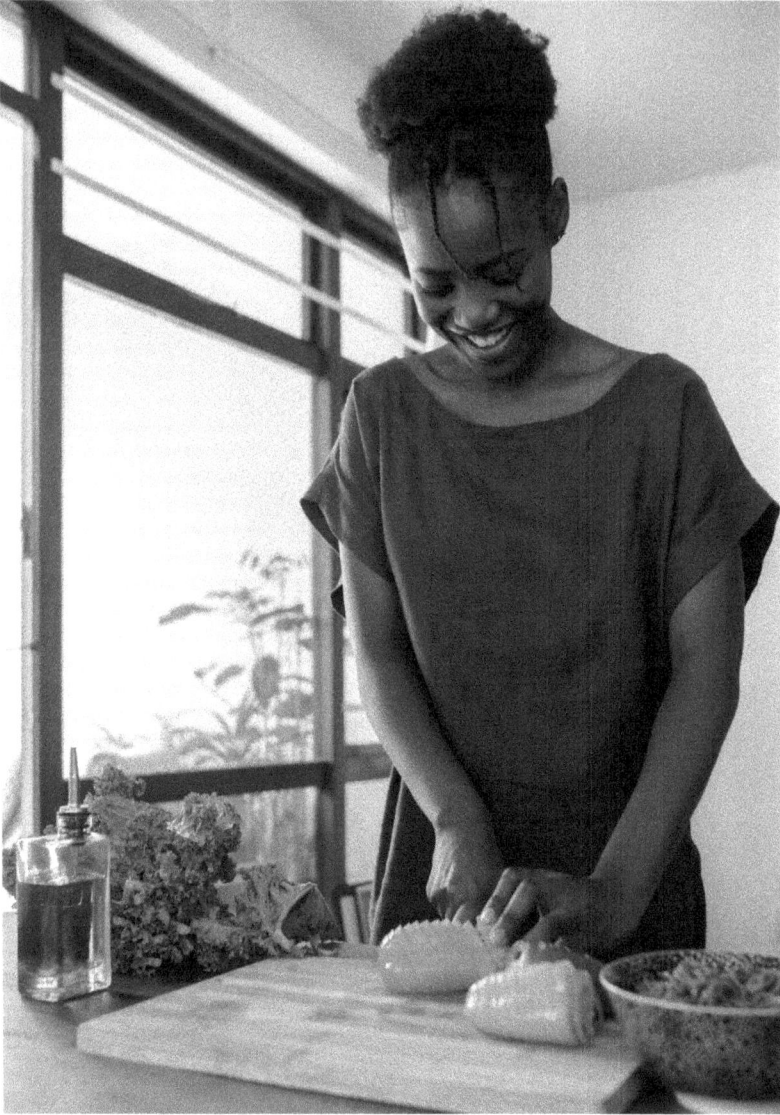

One of the very premises of nutrition is the principle that what we eat should provide something that the body is able to utilize. Anything we eat that the body cannot utilize is harmful.

Either something is nourishing to the body or it is harmful because anything the body cannot use must simply be eliminated as quickly as possible so that it does not interfere with the living processes. And anything that the body does not use and considers harmful or a foreign entity then requires a lot of energy for the body to attempt to neutralize or eliminate or both. Much of the 'food' we ingest is very difficult to eliminate and causes mucus and irritation which leads to cellular damage and other problems.

This is mentioned because food that has been subjected to the heat of a frying pan or an oven has been destroyed or deranged. The molecular bonds change with exposure to fire and these changes in the bonds of the food material render it much less nutritionally valuable and often it is actually harmful.

The human body can receive calories from cooked foods but does not recognize cooked food as a legitimate food. In fact consuming cooked foods is so foreign to our body that it often creates an immune system response revealing that it perceives a threat to the vital domain.

When the chemistry of a food source is transformed by fire or heat the changes effected make the food no longer valuable for human consumption. We will explore this in more detail in the chapter dedicated to Raw vs Cooked Food.

Although there is no nutrition we don't die very quickly eating cooked foods because primarily we need calories not nutrition. We need calories for fuel far more than we need nutritional factors such as vitamins and this is evidenced by how many people eat almost entirely a diet of cooked foods and still live many years.

CHAPTER 11

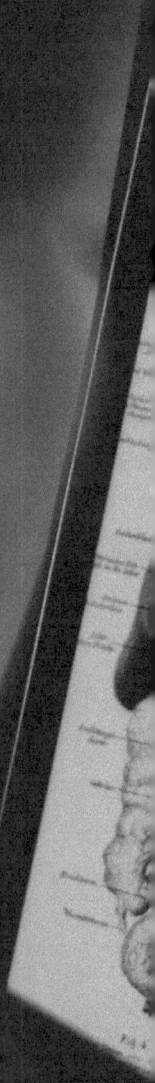

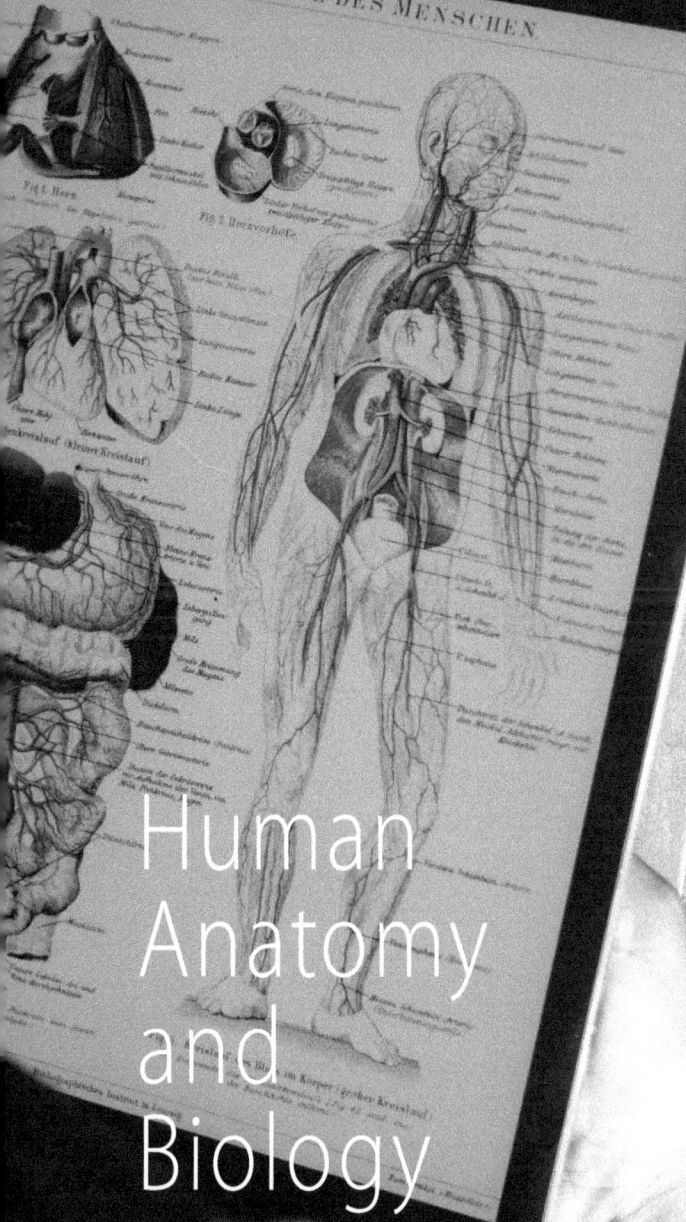

Human Anatomy and Biology

As we look at human anatomy and physiology and as we look at our closest genetic relatives on the planet we observe that we share a very similar anatomical design.

Comparative anatomy is the science that shows animals with similar digestive structures eat similar foods. This is a law of nature that has no exceptions. Certain animals have digestive systems are designed exclusively for flesh (the carnivore class), others only for grasses and leaves (the herbivore class), others for only fruit (the frugivore class) and those which have systems designed to assimilate all types of food (the omnivore class).

Almost all of us humans have grown up with the idea that we are members of the omnivore category and thus are designed to eat all classes of foods. *This is one of the biggest fallacies that leads to many serious errors in diet and this in turn is the cause of a great percentage of our diseases and symptoms.*

The analysis that deems humans to be omnivores is not an analysis at all, but rather is a product of retrofitting our science to our cultural patterns. Observing that certain modern cultures eat lots of meat and eggs and cheese has led scientists to incorrectly conclude that we as a species are omnivores and then to create a large library of factual sounding scientific literature to support the false belief in order to validate our cultural patterns of eating.

What does not seem to be considered is that we humans are by far the sickest species on the planet. In fact, no other species on earth gets sick and suffers from degenerative diseases to the extent that we do. These types of disease results are never seen in nature because wild animals eat according to their biology and anatomy. They also eat their foods 100% raw and they exercise as they go about their daily business every single day without exception.

When we go to a zoo we see the sign on the cages that reads, 'Do NOT Feed the Animals' and this sign is placed for a very important reason. The sign is there always in front of the most important animals that are valuable and not allowed to get sick. Veterinarians that work at the zoo and are responsible for animals know that diet is the key factor in maintaining the health of an animal.

Thus, the protocol that ensures the best health of animals relates to the absolute perfect regulation of the diet of the animal as per its anatomy. Veterinarians understand very well that the fastest way to sicken an animal is to feed it food that it was not designed to eat.

This point cannot be overstated because it lies at the heart of what is wrong with the modern medical paradigm that does not recognize the relationship between diet and disease in humans. We humans who play the role of directors of zoological parks worldwide know that for every species on earth the key to health is a proper natural diet based on digestive anatomy and structure of the specific animal.

But there seems to be a belief that humans are an exception. According to this almost unspoken belief we humans are not related to nature and are not subject to the laws of nature regarding diet like every other species. Apparently we do not have a specific diet like every single animal on earth. As mentioned earlier our culture seems to think that diet for humans is a matter of opinion rather than a matter of science as it is for all other organisms on this planet without exception.

Humans may be able to survive eating omnivorously for a while but humans are not omnivores in an optimal natural environment. We are not omnivores even though we can survive for some time eating a mix of foods and even as we take pharmaceuticals and live a sedentary life. But only for a while and then often we hit the wall of the laws of nature that we tried to break but we found that instead it was ourselves that broke.

People can survive for a while eating like an omnivore but surviving is not the same as thriving and nobody heals disease or has a powerful immune system without respecting what kind of species they are.

How do we know that we are not omnivores? Well one thing is that omnivores when they are without food for a short time will begin to simply eat each other. No matter how hungry a human family gets the human mother or father will not eat their children. This is how omnivores behave without exception. Omnivores are pigs and bears and dogs and humans do not resemble these creatures.

Humans are certainly not carnivores. That is very obvious. Our system has nothing in common with the digestive anatomy and our behavior patterns could not be more different from that of a carnivore like a wild cat which sleeps 20 hours a day due to eating large amounts of protein. Carnivores have digestive systems designed for flesh and the flesh is eaten without being cooked and very soon after the kill. Some carnivores don't even wait for the animal to die before they start to eat it. Humans would not readily do that.

Humans are also not herbivores as many people mistakenly suggest. I even see experts in the field of plant nutrition referring to humans casually as herbivores.

Humans are quite far from being herbivores. We do not resemble cows, giraffes, deer or any of the ungulates. We do not have multiple stomachs and thus we are unable to extract nutrition from grasses or leaves as do herbivores. We are unable to break down cellulose and we do not spend our entire waking life eating and re-chewing partially digested plant matter. The label of herbivore is almost, but not quite, as far off as the label of carnivore.

So, if we are not omnivores, carnivores or herbivores what are we? What is left? Most people do not know that there is an entire other class of organisms that are called *frugivores*.

Frugivores are fruit eaters and are represented on earth in the great apes like mountain gorilla, orangutan, chimpanzee, gibbon and humans. We are a member of a family of great apes that is designed to eat almost exclusively fruit. As mentioned previously, the author worked for many years at a primate zoo in South Florida and observed the veterinarians feeding these great apes every single day.

What were they fed so that they remained in perfect health? 100% fruit!

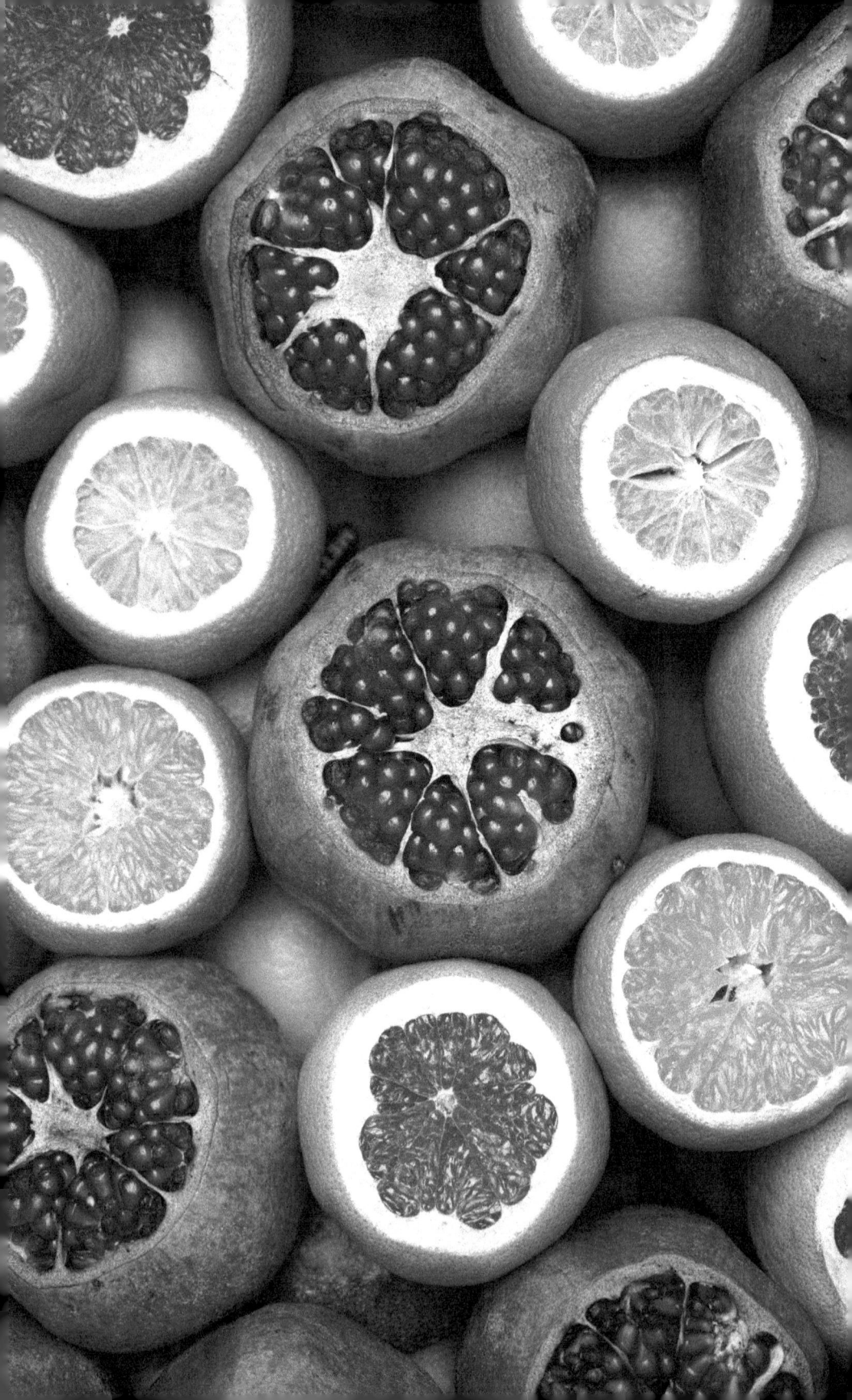

This is why the more fruit we eat as humans the healthier we become and the better we feel. Eating according to biology has its advantages! Some of our most powerful protocols for helping people to resolve their health issues involve putting people temporarily on a 100% fruit diet so that their bodies can turn on as they were programmed and heal.

Once healed the person would want to continue to eat as much fruit as possible while potentially moving into a more relaxed posture with some other plant foods.

In sum, it is that simple, we are designed to eat fruit. If that is not enough to convince you, try this: take a piece of raw meat with no seasoning, no salt, no smoke, no sauce, nothing but the meat alone. At room temperature break it apart, close your eyes and smell it. I mean really smell the dead flesh before you imagine to take a bite. Does that sound appealing? Now, take a bite of a banana or strawberry or mango or other fresh fruit. Which one tastes like food to you?

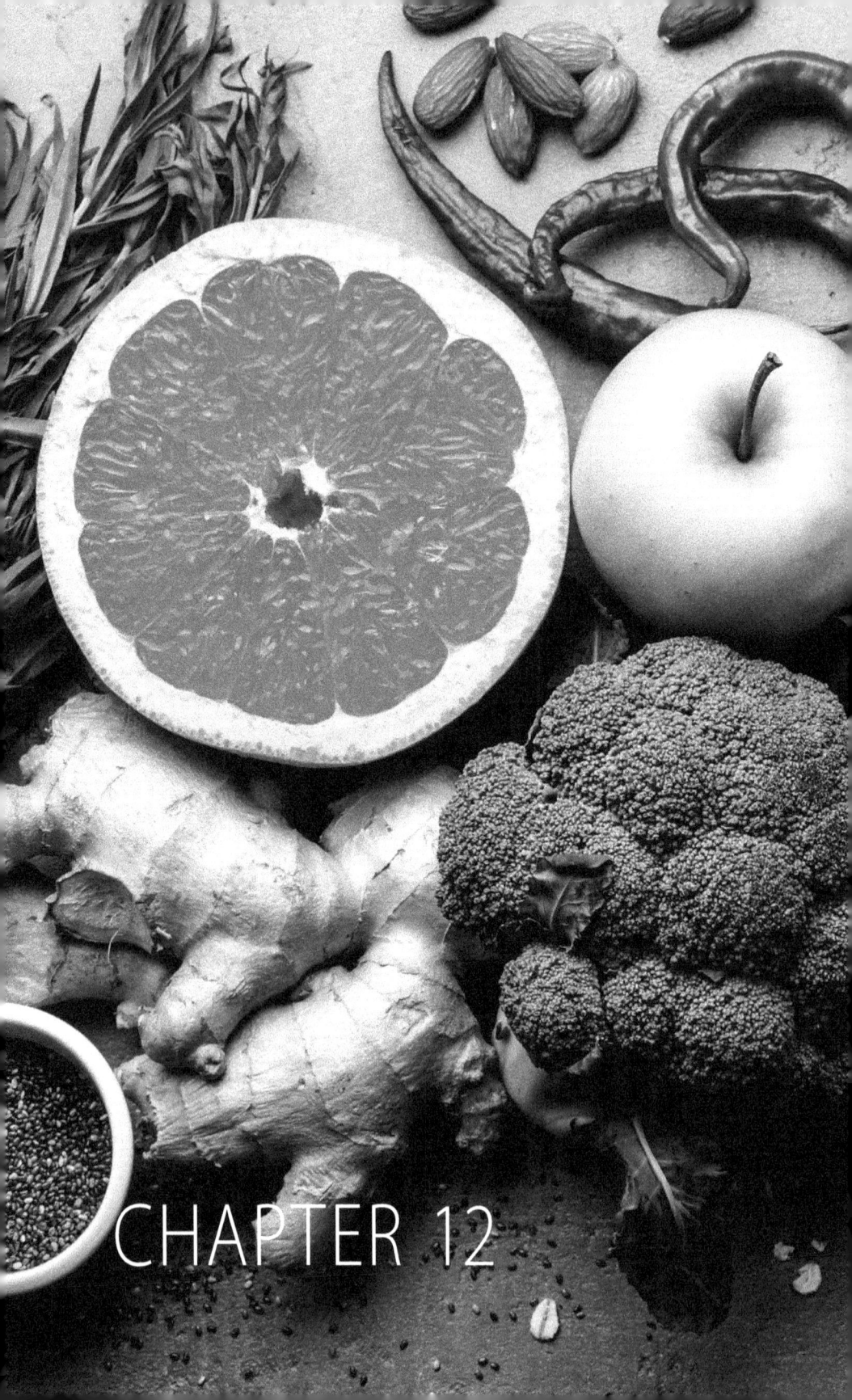

CHAPTER 12

Raw vs
Cooked
Food

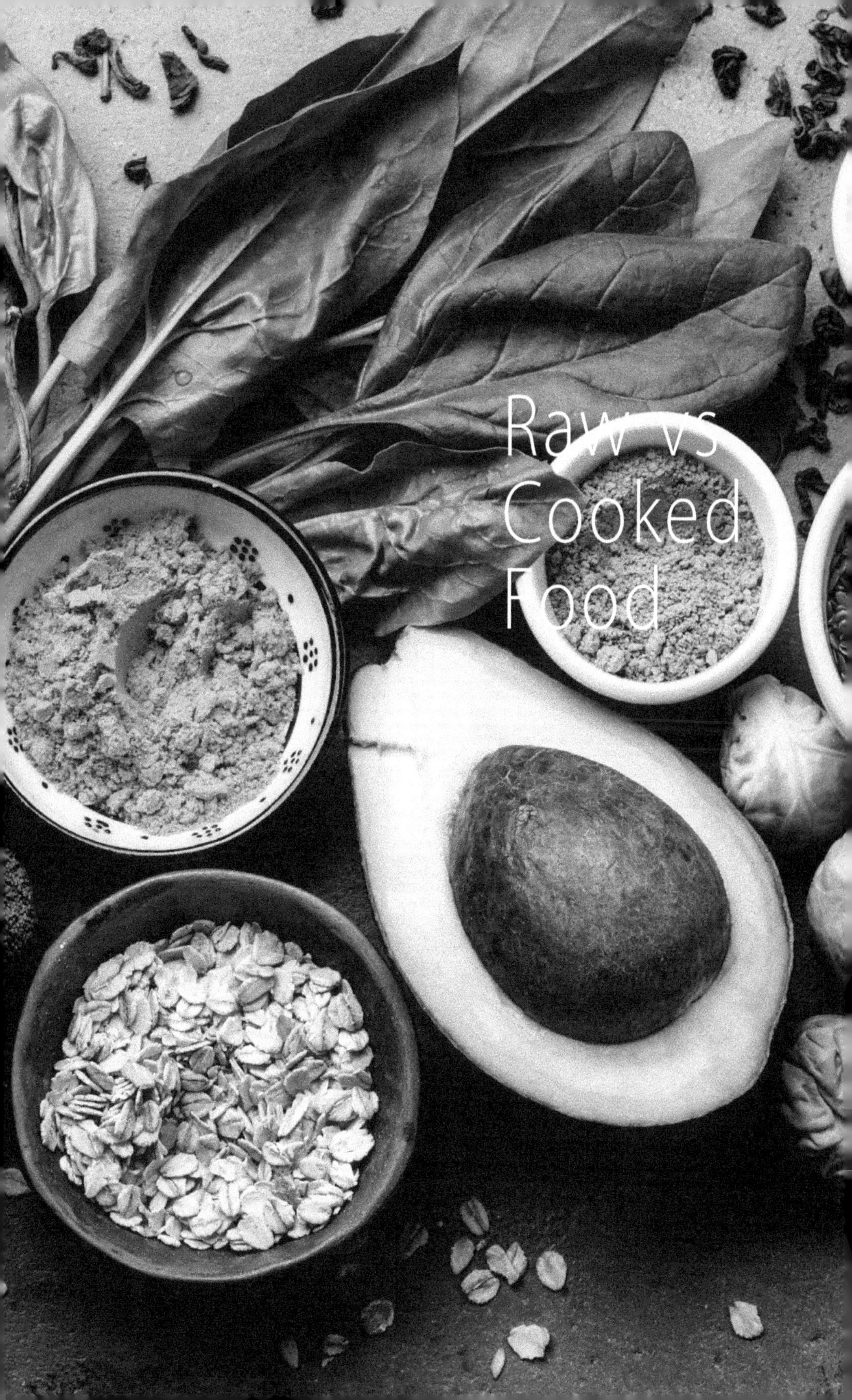

It would be very challenging to find a subject that is so simple and yet so misunderstood by so many people. It is nothing short of astounding how few people are able to appreciate this subject. The subject I am referring to is the principle that food should not be cooked.

Perhaps it stems from the cultural obstacle of questioning the way our mothers fed us as a child or perhaps because it is because cooked food can taste so good, but for whatever reason this one concept has escaped the grasp of most, including many experts.

Let me first say that I am not suggesting that regular people reading this book shift to 100% raw vegan diet. Nevertheless, I am suggesting that it is the ideal and that if we are confronted with a health challenge that it indeed should be employed in order for that issue to be resolved as quickly and effectively as possible.

When we have a health challenge and we have symptoms of some variety it is a clear message from the body. The body is not sending a message asking for pharmaceutical poisons. The message the body sends when symptoms arise is 'this is not an ideal environment for best health and that something needs to change'. And, when the body expresses symptoms or disease manifestations it is very important that we heed this message and align all our activities to nature's anatomical design. This means not eating foods that have been destroyed by fire.

So, this is a very simple rule. The rule is followed by every single living organism on Earth, without one single exception. We are talking about the rule of not destroying your food before you eat it. No other organism on earth destroys or degrades its food source with high heat and fire before ingestion.

This cannot be overstated. As we look at the natural kingdom of life forms we observe very easily and absolutely that all organisms consume their food in an uncooked state. Fire has only been very recently mastered and used in the kitchens of humanity – perhaps only the last 10 thousand years at the most. But, we have been in this Homo sapiens form for approximately 1 million years give or take. That means that even humans have for the vast majority of existence consumed foods without cooking them.

Having been a student of science and philosophy I have always had a foundation in the philosophy of logic. I have always sought to use the smell test of logic before requiring my brain to think on a subject more in depth.

So, let us ask ourselves logically speaking this question: *if all organisms on earth feed in a certain manner, in this case eating uncooked foods, what are the chances that the one species being considered apart would be the exception?*

What are the chances logically that we are an exception to the laws of nature? In my view the logical answer is basically none. There is basically no chance whatsoever that we as humans are somehow not subject to the same law as every other earthling.

Cooked food behaves like a poison in your body. Immune system responses are reported after we ingest cooked foods. These reports suggest that the body is producing leukocytes (white blood cells) when we eat cooked foods which means that the body does not recognize cooked foods as something that belongs in the human body. White blood cells are created by the body only when it is confronted by substances that are foreign and need to be eliminated or neutralized.

Fire destroys biological life, changes chemistry and electromagnetic bonds, and leaves a result that is quite different from the original unburned material. When this gets applied to foods it means that almost all of the nutritional factors that made the food valuable are no longer available. When a vegetable for example is cooked, the vitamins and minerals and essential fatty acids and amino acids are all changed into a form that is much less useful or even, in fact, useless to the body.

Raw foods contain life force and vital nutritional elements that sustain life. Dead or cooked foods are barren of both of these. When we start eating more and more raw foods, especially fruit, we begin to feel a different level of energy. It is common sense to some degree that when we eat foods that have energy we get energy and when we eat foods devoid of energy our overall energy levels lower.

Eating cooked foods also wastes lots of energy. So much of our energy is wasted in the digestive system as the body attempts to break down cooked foods that have been made unrecognizable to the intelligence in the stomach. One reason why many people are ill is that they are totally drained energetically from living for years without proper energetics entering the body.

Related to this subject, this is the basic reason why fasting on water or juices is such a healing practice. Energy that is not being misused in the attempted digestion of cooked and coagulated foods can be redirected to the cleansing and healing of the body.

When we eat as few cooked foods as possible we are able to get a large degree of those benefits also because raw foods like fruits are very easy on our digestive system. Raw vegetables are not as easy to digest and must be chewed very well and can be juiced if desired but fruits are far superior. This is due to the fact as discussed earlier that we are not herbivores and vegetables while healthy are not our primary food in an ideal environment as that award belongs to the great fruit kingdom.

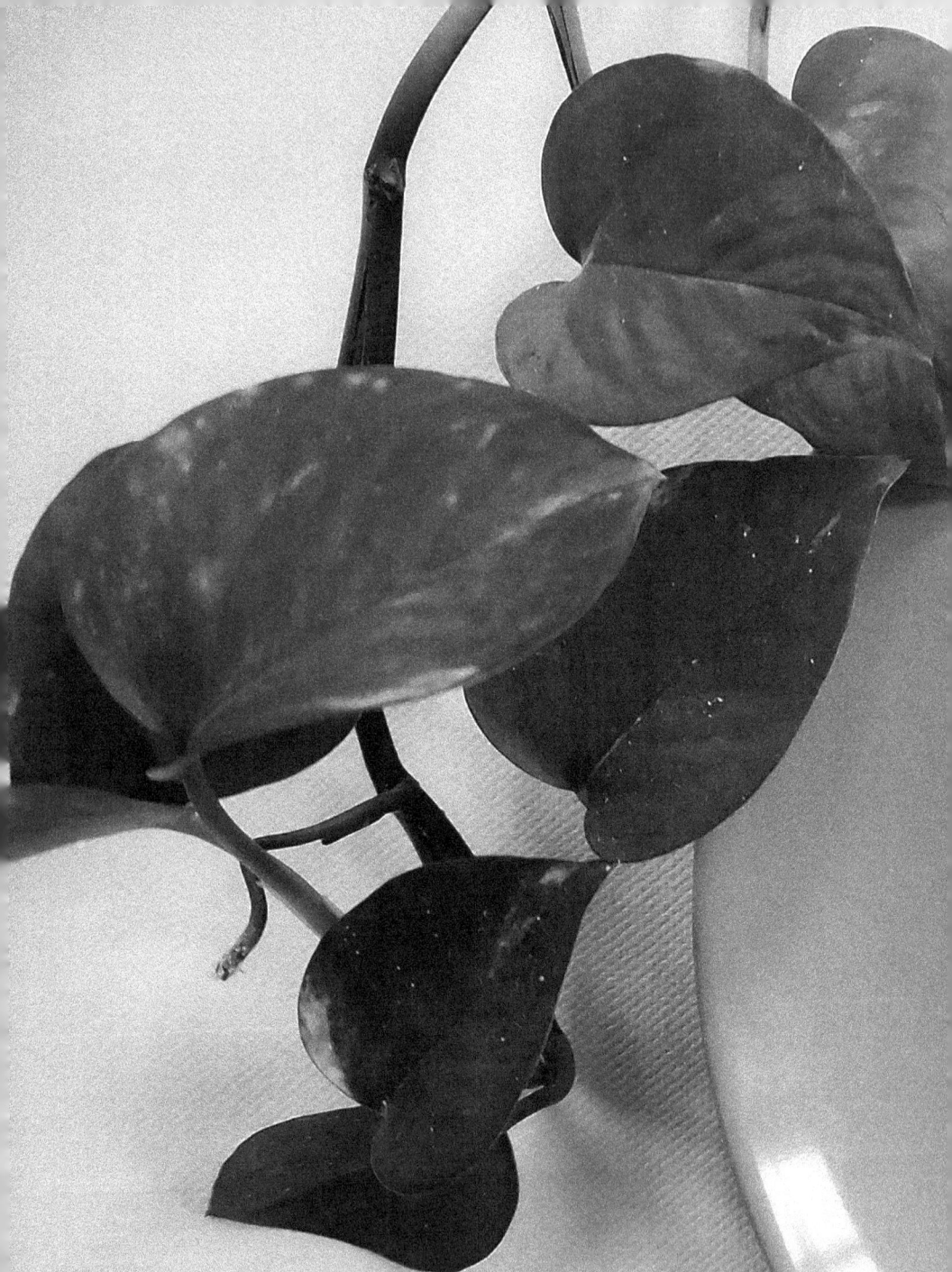

CHAPTER 13

The
Spectrum
of Diets

VEGAN

One of the most common questions after reading all this material and more is of course *'What am I to eat?'*

The most basic answer is that you should eat in the best way that you can sustain in a long-term capacity. A diet that you can accomplish realistically is the key. Making a declaration that you will only eat fruit for the rest of your life is not realistic for most of us and creating an overenthusiastic goal may only lead to disappointment and resentment at the process. It is very important that you are able to sustain an intelligent way of eating for a very long time as opposed to being radically perfect for too long and then relapsing back to poor choices.

Having said that there is a spectrum of truth relating to what humans are designed to eat which is also the spectrum of the diets that heal humans from their disease conditions the fastest.

Here is the spectrum:

The very best diets in order of power to heal and strengthen the immune system are:

1) 100% Fruit

2) 100% Raw Vegan/Plant Based with a focus on fruits primarily

3) 100% Raw Vegan/Plant Based without emphasizing fruit

4) 100% Vegan/Plant Based with a very large percentage of fruit and raw food

5) 100% Vegan without focus on raw foods

There are no really good diets after that because of course from there we move into the realm of the vegetarian who eats eggs and milk. For all vegetarians and omnivores and even self-proclaimed carnivores, the fewer animal products they consume and the more fresh fruit they consume the better their diet will become.

Due to the spectrum of nature dietary law it is important to realize that even very small steps in the right direction are actually large. A person at the bottom of the dietary spectrum eating lots of meat and fish and who decides to try for a few weeks to be vegetarian will have accomplished a very important step even if they are not trying to get to the raw food levels. One step at a time and without any sense of deprivation is the only way to relate to food.

There are no absolutes to diet except for the people who are eating 100% fruit and that is often not realistic. Best is to see clearly the fact that everything is relative in the dietary world and do the best possible without self-criticism or self-judgement. .

One of the most common mistakes we make is the self-suggestion that if we only eat something healthy once that it won't make a difference really. This is the same false suggestion that people make about exercise and it is very dangerous because it leads to us doing nothing. The fact is that small steps are huge because they get us onto the positive feedback loop mentioned earlier which is the key to success.

Also please remember that if you can simply eliminate some of the worst things you eat and replace them with better versions or more fruits even just once, you have made a monumental step in the right direction. Every single bit counts!

CHAPTER 14

Happiness
piece of c

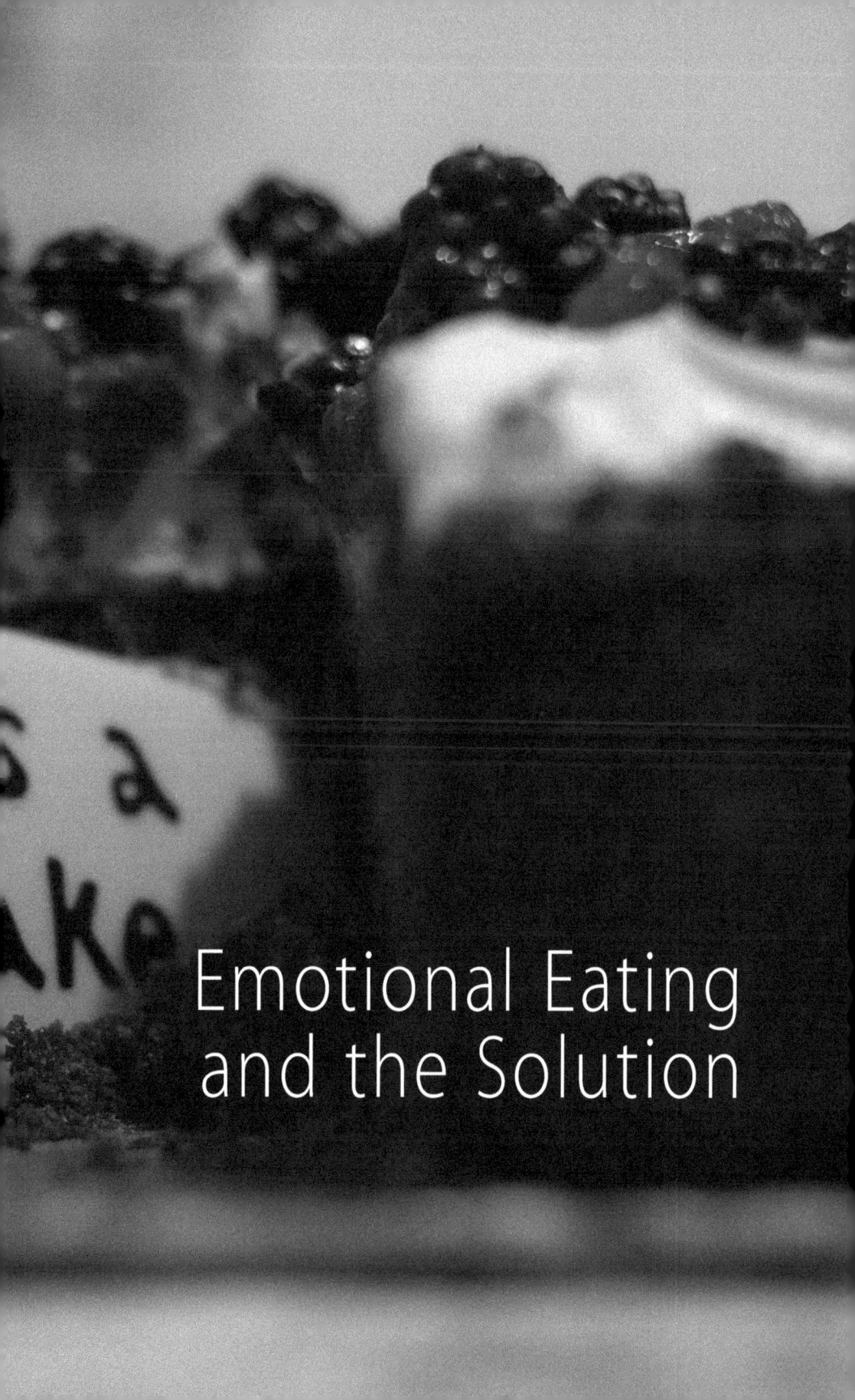

Emotional Eating
and the Solution

One of the greatest challenges we face regarding food is the tendency to use eating to deal with stress or a variety of emotional issues.

Many of us have turned to consuming junk food in a misguided effort to make us feel a little better. This is called emotional eating and must be recognized as a toxic pattern of behavior to be transcended.

Unfortunately, there is a strong correlation between depression and emotional eating. As people feel depressed and dejected they are also feeling an emptiness which seems to be uniquely filled by poor food choices. This creates the negative feedback cycle mentioned earlier because feeling bad and eating bad reinforce each other and result in a bad situation becoming worse.

Comfort food is another name describing this type of food which is more about our emotional needs than our biological requirements.

So what is the solution? How do we transcend or overcome the tendency towards emotional eating?

First, practices like meditation and yoga transform consciousness so that the feelings of emptiness are minimized or eliminated. If you have never meditated or practiced yoga, you may be skeptical about this approach but I strongly encourage you to take a leap of faith and participate in these activities that have been scientifically proven to change the way your brain functions by giving you greater levels of consciousness from which to see.

Second, don't be too hard on yourself. Understand, that we can't avoid emotional eating 100% of the time because our minds are very comforted by eating certain foods in certain situations. However if you are aware that emotional eating is sometimes unavoidable you can simply select a more healthy version of the food and greatly mitigate any effects of eating poorly.

But by choosing the vegan cheeseburger or the coconut milk ice cream we get the experience we feel comforted by while being orders of magnitude better than the original version.

As long as it is done with awareness, emotional eating is not a problem per se. The awareness that you have chosen to eat emotionally and the selection of a more intelligent version of your emotional food of choice are the two ways to mitigate the downside.

It is very important never to criticize yourself while enjoying an emotional meal but rather to truly and fully enjoy what you are eating in the moment. As long as you give yourself full permission to eat things you want and you really enjoy them, it is likely you will not crave them as much since cravings often come from that which we feel deprived of.

CHAPTER 15

Your Results: 'Be Your Own Scientist'

Do not take our word for anything you read in this book. How do you know what we are saying is true? Perhaps what you are reading makes sense to you intellectually but that is not enough. There is only one way to verify truth...*experience!*

A person whose body is functioning at 40% of its natural capacity has no way of imagining what it feels like to live in a body that is fully healthy and in harmony with nature. Thus only experience can deliver the real truth.

Only when a person who was previously functioning sub-optimally, with low energy and or illnesses experiences for *themselves* the energizing and immune system boosting effects of the Five Fundamental Factors will they realize what has been missing in their lives.

Be like a scientist who is testing a hypothesis and give yourself 30 days at least to make your own determination. Make the 100% change to whatever diet you choose on the spectrum and do it for some significant time like the 30 days mentioned and then see for yourself!

Once you have the actual experience of what happens when your body is fed according to biology, exercises daily, rests well, is aware of the power of mind, and lives more organically then you will truly know and probably wonder why it took so long to learn these simple lessons.

Take it as an experiment for the sake of science and then analyze the results and if you are not pleased you are always free to revert back to previous operating patterns and at least you know you gave it a try. You have nothing to lose and everything to gain.

So, set your calendar for four weeks and determine that you will avoid all animal foods and eat as much fruit as you can. Exercise each day and begin a short meditation practice. Get a bit of extra sleep, start avoiding common chemical exposures in your daily life and then just wait a very short time for the results to come in. You are the scientist as well the experiment so the results will stand revealed quite clearly.

CHAPTER 16

Dairy

There are many interrelated reasons to avoid consuming dairy. First and foremost, it is a violation of nature. Second, it is poorly digested. Third, it has proven serious adverse effects on the body. We will discuss all of this below, but, simply put, dairy is not food for humans, except for infants consuming human milk.

We humans are mammals and by definition, all mammals share these traits:

1) Warm-blooded; 2) Hair; 3) Live birth; 4) Lactation mammary glands milk drinking infant; and 5) Weaning process.

The last one is the most important. Mammals drink the milk produced by their mother after birth for a certain period of time that varies among species but always comes to an end at some point very early in the life of the young mammal. After the specified period of time the young mammal will begin to reject their mother's milk and eat the foods that the species eats.

As an interesting aside, human milk is not a simple substance and contains a complex mixture of biological growth factors that vary over time to meet an infant's needs as it matures. The point here is that milk is specifically designed for infants and further engineered based on the infant's stage of development.

More importantly, no animal in nature consumes the milk of another animal. And, as discussed above no adult animal on earth consumes its mother's milk. Substances like cow's milk and goat's milk are just not natural food for anything except cows and goats. It might be obvious that the growth factors needed to produce a baby cow that are present in cow's milk are far from what is required to produce a baby human. Dairy products are promoted by large multinational food companies trying to sell something for a profit and are not agents of health and wellness as they advertise their calcium or protein.

Studies not sponsored by big dairy producers show that dairy is not at all healthy. Various studies have revealed that casein, the protein found in milk, is linked with the growth of tumors. Books like *The China Study* also document quite clearly the links between casein consumption and cancer.

Studies also show that milk causes you to produce excessive amounts of mucus in your gut, sinus area and lungs. This is very troublesome because mucus blocks functioning and specifically your gut is a center of your immune system. As most know from experience the sinus cavity can become infected from mucus stagnation all caused from dairy.

Lactose, the primary sugar found in dairy, does not break down in adults. Adult mammals do not produce the enzyme lactase, which results in the lactose not being broken down correctly, which in turn leads to fermentation, gas and damage to cells.

Another issue worthy of discussion is the relationship between dairy consumption and osteoporosis. This subject is almost criminally misrepresented by modern nutritionists and perpetuated even by most medical doctors. Beginning in the 1950s many nutritionists and doctors have promoted the idea that since bones are made mostly of calcium and we want strong bones, we must increase our levels of calcium in milk to increase our bone strength.

The thinking was that since dairy foods have lots of calcium that consuming dairy foods like milk were effectively a healthy dietary choice. Marketing of dairy products by large corporate producers has focused on and promoted the belief that calcium in dairy products prevent osteoporosis and promotes 'strong bones'.

Unfortunately, precisely the opposite is true. Although it is true that dairy foods have calcium the fact is that the consumption of dairy causes the adult body to lose more calcium that it can absorb because of the acidic nature of the dairy after being digested.

As we consume dairy or meats or anything acidic our body must neutralize the blood chemistry and keep it to a certain pH to prevent death from acidosis, and it accomplishes this goal by releasing alkaline calcium and magnesium ions from the vessels and the bones. As a result, the veins become compromised and varicose and the bones get weaker and porous and this is the condition known as 'osteoporosis'.

The real solution to bone density does not lie in consuming calcium from dairy or even processed supplement pills but rather from whole plant foods which are alkaline along with exercising and strength training of the physical body to stimulate bone density and regeneration.

In sum, the bottom line is that consuming dairy is not healthy and should be avoided by those wishing to experience wellbeing.

Can a person who consumes dairy be called a vegetarian? Not really because the dairy industry and veal industry are inextricably linked so anyone who drinks milk and cheese is causing the death of a baby animal automatically.

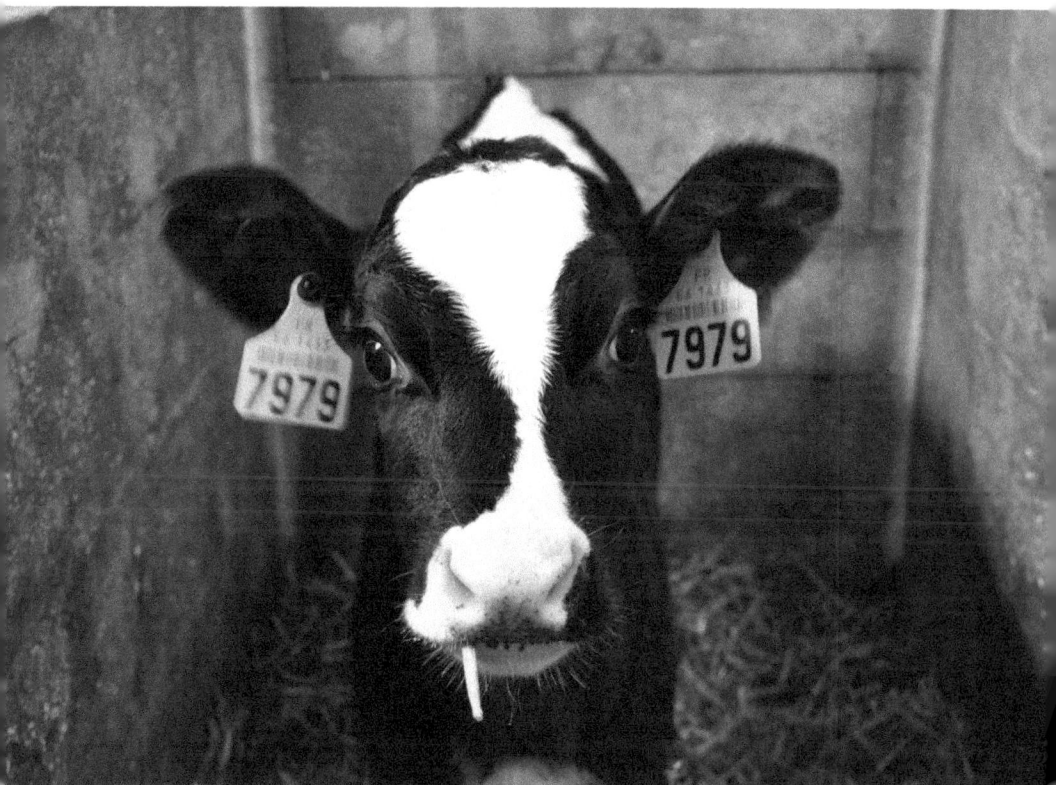

CHAPTER 17

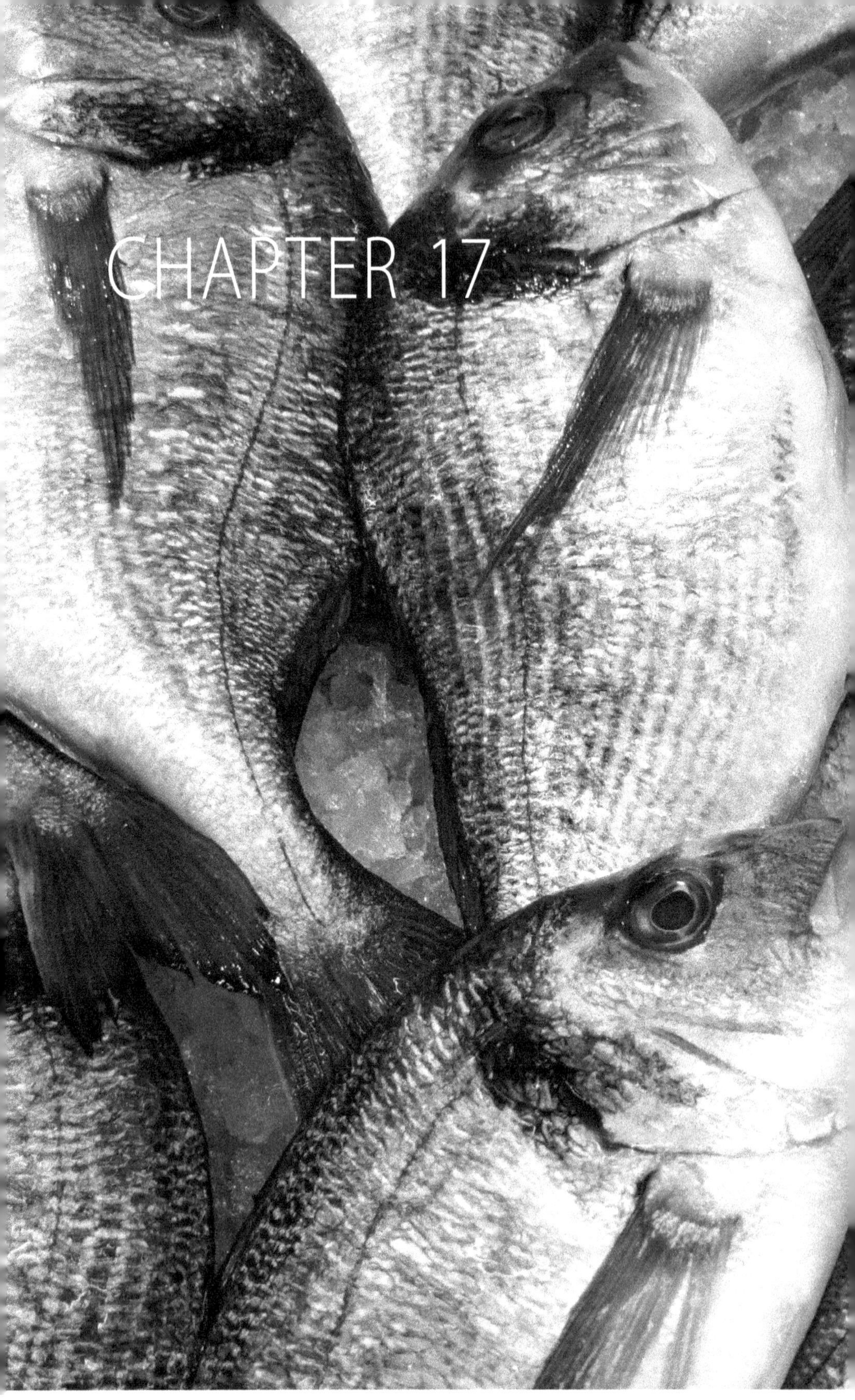

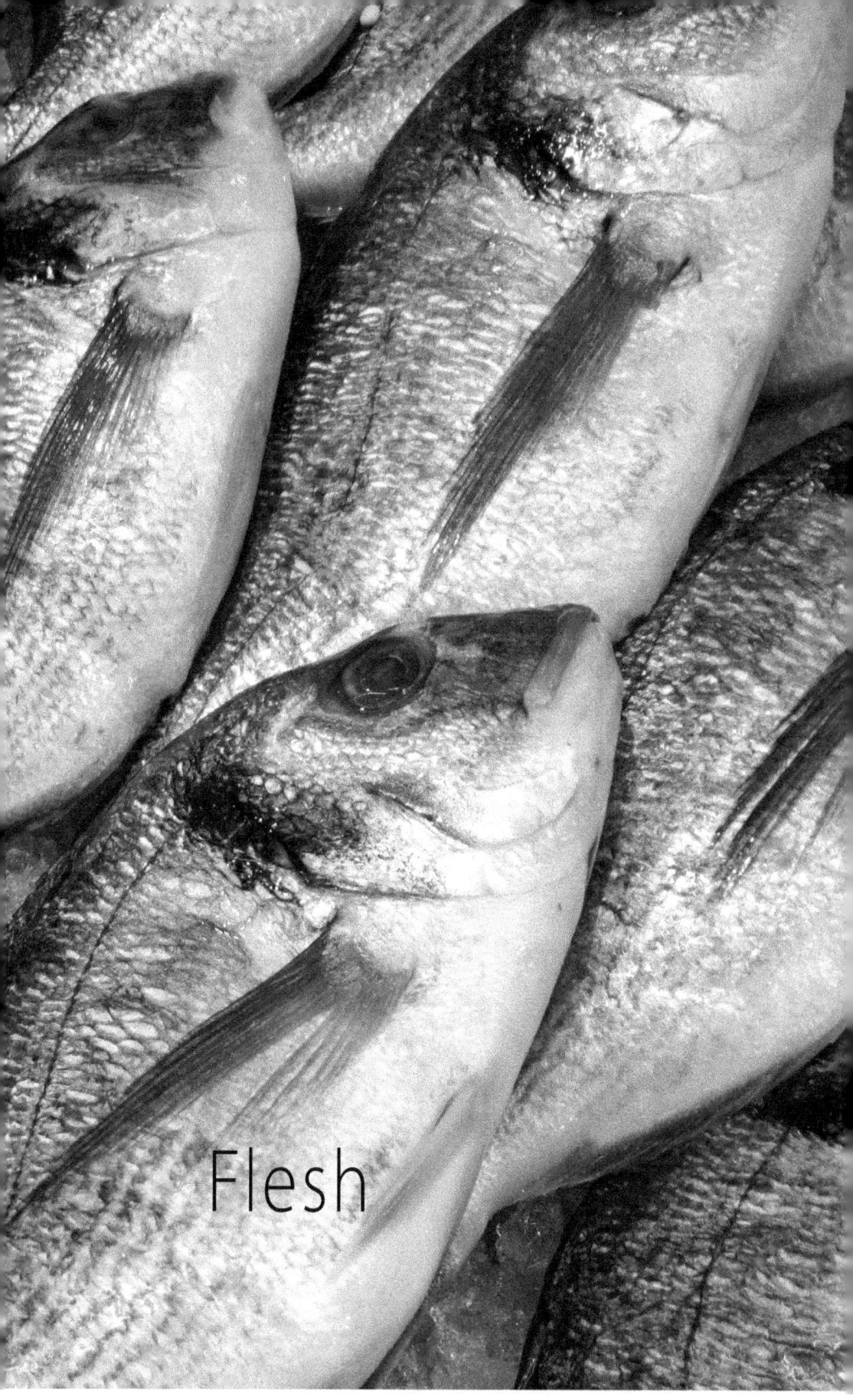

Flesh

Humans are members of the primate family known as great apes. All great apes have a similar anatomy and humans therefore share a digestive system structure with the other great apes. Our genetic relatives like the chimpanzee, bonobo, mountain gorilla, gibbon and orangutan, all have a digestive structure designed primarily to eat fruit, as do we.

As mentioned earlier the science of comparative anatomy dictates that in nature, animals that share a digestive structure also eat the same class of foods. The great apes are mostly fruit eaters and their digestive system is designed and dependent upon high levels of fiber, like that found in fruit and lacking in flesh, for proper functioning.

Unlike humans and the other great apes, animals that are designed to hunt are given the physical capacity to kill their prey. Without exception, nature provides the tools in the form of physical characteristics that can accomplish the killing. For example, eagles have the eyesight, wings and talons to kill snakes; and lions have the claws, strength and teeth to subdue large animals. These animals were born with these physical characteristics which enable them to survive and thrive in the wild. Wild animals do not have to buy or make the means with which they kill their prey.

Humans are simply not born with tools capable of killing the vast majority of what we consider to be our food. We are unable to catch almost any animal and we are unable to kill most animals with just our hands. Imagine a human trying to catch and kill a steer without weapons or tools. Or, imagine yourself trying to catch a bird. This fact offers some evidence to support the principle that we are not designed to eat flesh, since if we were, we would be armed and much more capable of killing any animal we eat, as true predators are.

A common question arises: *How can so many people eat so much flesh and survive if what this book is saying is true?*

Although human beings do not thrive on a diet that includes any significant amount of flesh foods, the human organism is unbelievably robust and able to survive while eating a very poor diet as long as calories are ingested. This is the reason that most people believe that humans are actually omnivores. However as mentioned earlier, just because we can survive eating an omnivorous diet does not make us omnivores. In fact it simply makes us animals that have their health compromised when eating omnivorously. Simply put, we severely compromise our long-term health by eating foods that our bodies are not designed to eat.

Omnivores are pigs and bears and dogs but not humans. We can eat these mixed diets but we can also pay a high price with our long-term health. Just because we can stuff a dead animal down our throats and live to tell the story does not make it something your body was designed to eat.

Eating omnivorously is to some degree imagining that you are living in such a harsh environment that fruit and plants don't grow! With the modern supermarket this is not the case so there is no reason to eat the inferior flesh and dairy foods when the superior fruits are available.

There is a prevailing belief that flesh food offers some nutritional benefit or that they have components that plants and fruits do not have. This is false. There is nothing nutritionally valuable in an animal that was not first in a plant that the animal ate.

The source of nutrition is always the plant kingdom. Even animals that eat other animals are just eating animals that got

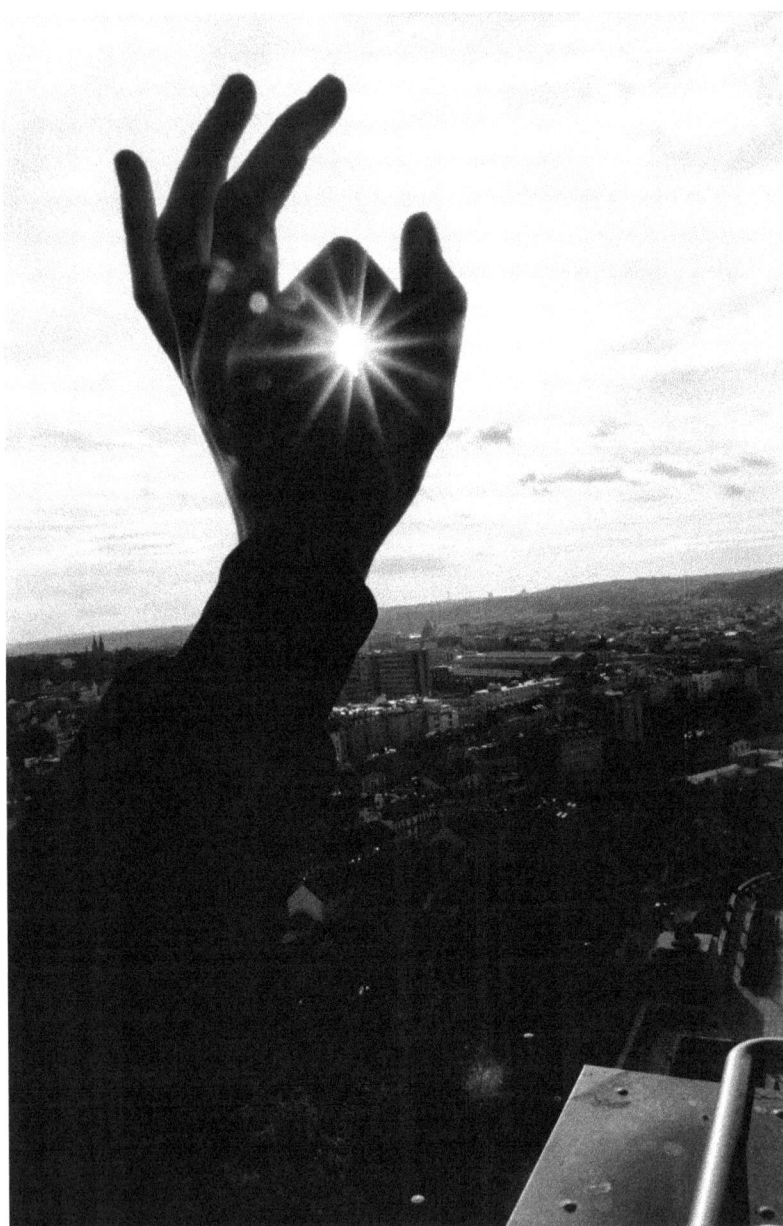

the original nutrition from the plant kingdom. The original energy that all life forms are ultimately assimilating is the energy of the sun.

The sun's energy fuels the entire planet and only the plant kingdom has direct access to it through the amazing process of photosynthesis. Solar energy is stored and incorporated into the plant kingdom. So, it is undeniable that plants are the best source of direct energy and of all food elements on earth, since they are *all* produced in the plant kingdom.

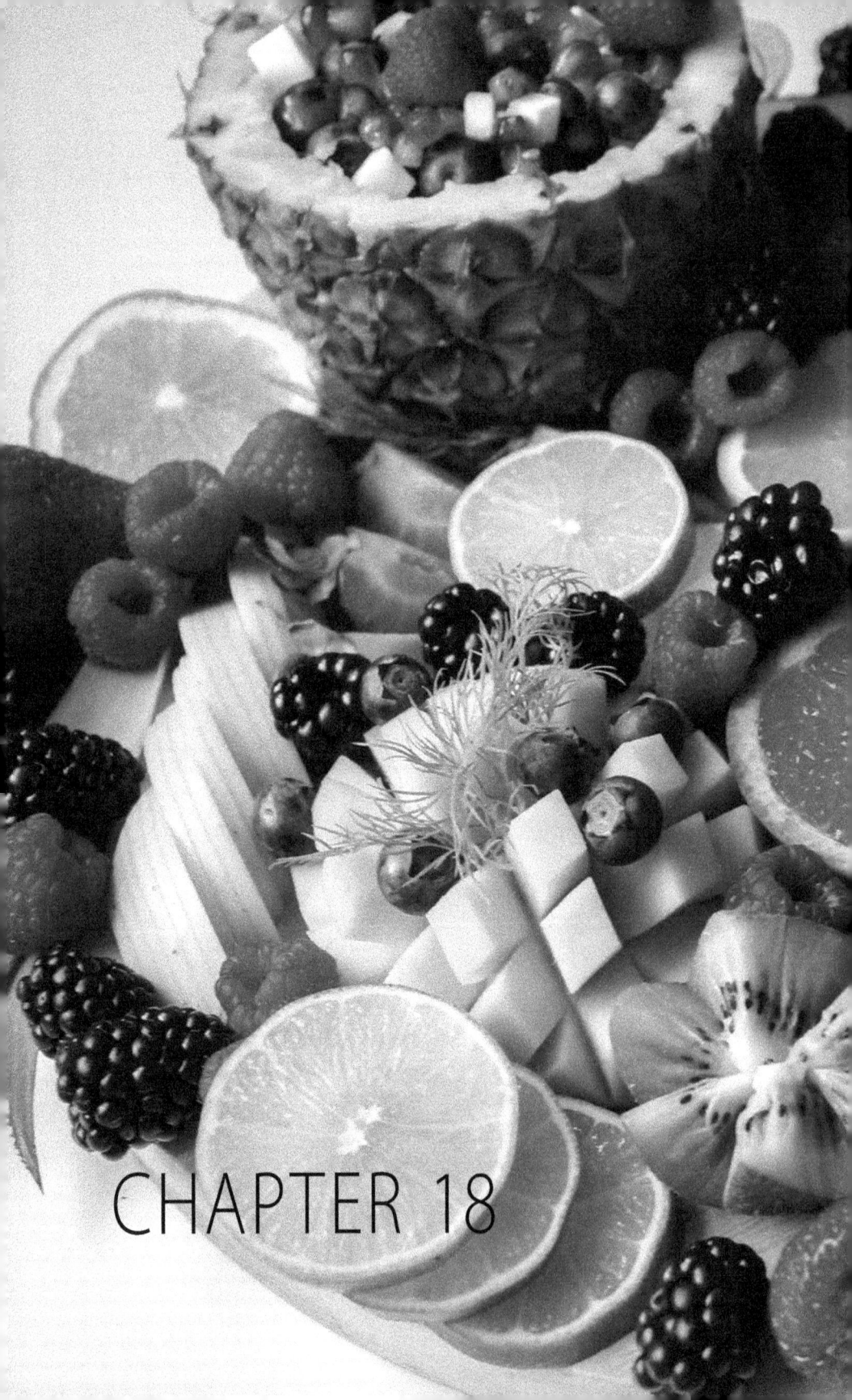

CHAPTER 18

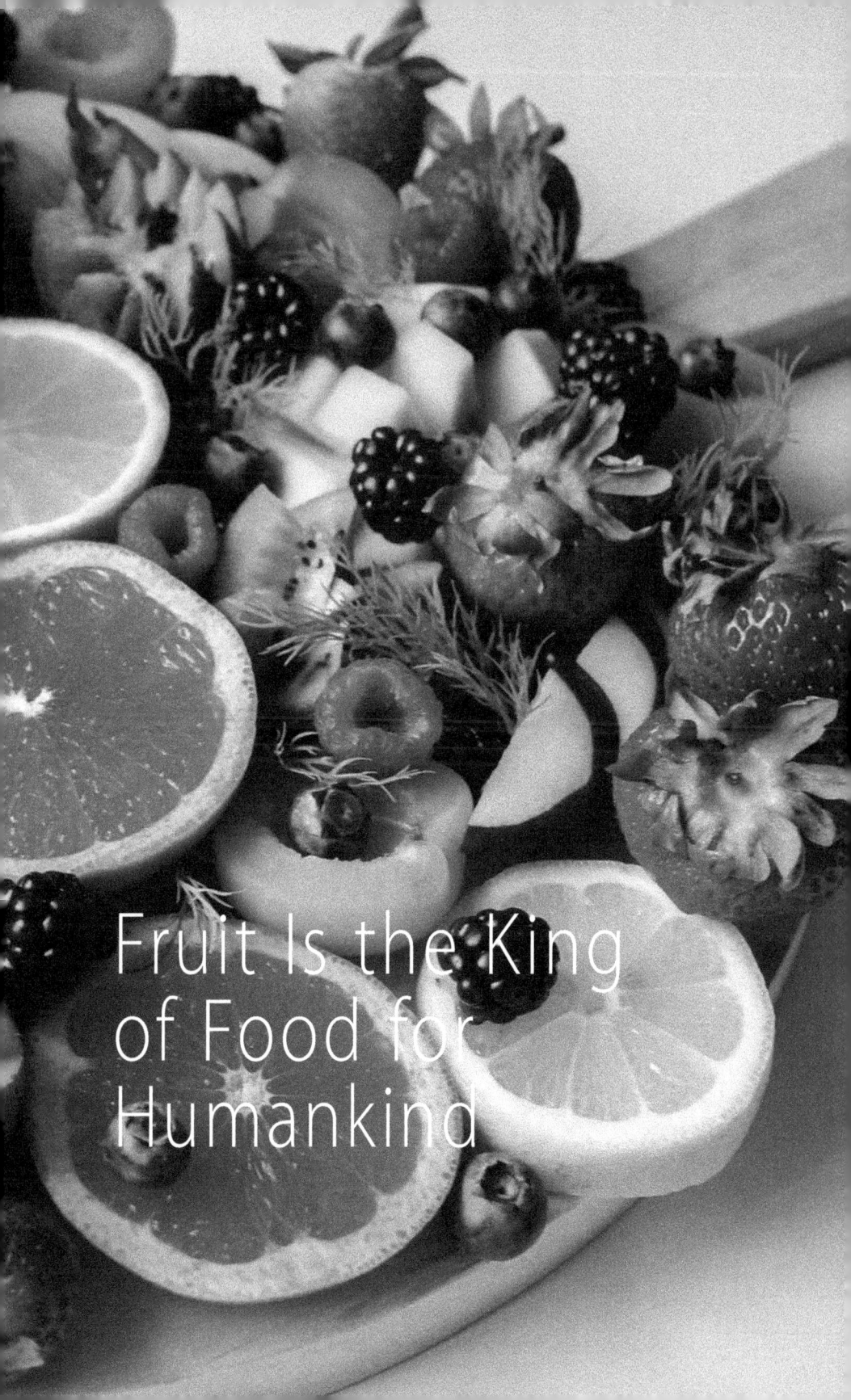

Fruit Is the King
of Food for
Humankind

Hippocrates, the father of Medicine put when he said, 'Let your *food* be your medicine and your medicine be your *food*'.

As primates, fruit is the key food for humans. Because as Hippocrates said *food is medicine*, fruit, being the best food source for humans is also the most effective and powerful way of helping to strengthen the immune system to experience health and vigor.

When we return to eating more fruit, which is the food most in alignment to our biology, our body begins to heal itself. Although the human body is a potent self-healing organism, it will only operate at full efficiency when certain conditions are met. One of the conditions for the body to work at full strength at healing is the consumption of almost entirely fruit for a certain period of time.

As earlier discussed, we share digestive anatomy with the great apes which means we are designed to eat similarly. Great apes in nature eat almost 100% fruits.

It is almost magical what occurs when we return to our natural diet. All manner of degenerative diseases can reverse themselves upon the application of a fruit-only dietary protocol.

Fruit has all the nutrition you need. Fruit also contains an electromagnetic energy that Eastern cultures refer to as 'chi' or 'prana' and which is considered to be more responsible for energizing the life within our bodies than the nutritional elements themselves.

This powerful electromagnetic energy in fruit is transferred to our bodies when eaten. It is not inaccurate to visualize that a person is swallowing little charging packs. Every time a person eats fruit they are literally charging the body with energy.

Fruit is a superfood – All fruits are superfoods, not just the ones that have been well marketed. Fruits are superfoods because they all contain a variety of compounds known as phytonutrients or phytochemicals. These compounds are not well understood and not well studied because they cannot be isolated and still retain their properties. In other words, they simply cannot be studied with the standard approach of scientific laboratory testing. However there is enough evidence to support the belief that fruits contain powerful anti-mutagenic and anti-tumor and antioxidant properties.

Fruit is alkaline – Alkalizing foods such as fruit are beneficial and most people these days are aware of the importance of eating more of an alkaline diet. The pH scale describes how acid or alkaline a substance is on scale of 1 to 14 with 7 being neutral and under 7 being acidic. Most fruits are alkaline to the blood after digestion. Even citrus, which appears to be acid, is alkaline after the digestive process. So then one of the best ways to keep the body alkaline is to eat as much fruit as we can!

Fruit is hydrating – Fruit prevents dehydration which causes cell damage and deterioration. Fruit is the perfect food with its combination of hydration and electrolytes. The water in fruit is pure and the quality of fruits is astringent which means fruits are powerful cleansers of the blood vessels. Fruit also cleanses mucus from the whole system which promotes health and vitality.

Fruit is antioxidant – The oxidation process is also called the burning process and occurs when molecules gets exposed to oxygen which has a corrosive effect. In metal this is called rusting. In living cells this same type of oxidation is the source of cellular damage as oxygen is a very powerful transformer of chemical bonds. Cellular damage is caused by oxidation by what are known as free radicals. Free radicals are missing an electron and are aggressively seeking to strip electrons from other atoms to complete their electron ring. Antioxidants are molecules with extra hydrogen ions which counter the harmful effects of the free radicals. Fruits are the highest in antioxidants of all foods.

Fruit is attractive and delicious – Why people do not eat more fruit is a bit of a mystery as we are naturally attracted to eating fruit. It is not a coincidence that children love fruit. After all, most fruit is delicious!

Also, fruit is colorful and bright colors are naturally pleasing to our senses and attract our eyes. We naturally have an interest in colorful foods because in nature we associate colors with fruits which means high nutrition. This fact has been used against us all by producers of colorful candies like 'm and m's' or 'skittles' or colored sprinkles on ice cream. They all appeal to our senses and tempt us subconsciously to eat them. This is also true of the hamburger or sub sandwich advertisements that are filled with colorful fresh vegetables like lettuce and tomato. Therefore although colorful vegetables are appealing in these ads we are also bombarded with images of foods that we should be avoiding.

Fruit *does not* have too much sugar – One of the most pervasive myths circulating over the last many years is the false idea that fruit has too much sugar. This could not be more misinformed. Not all sugars are equal and using the same word to describe vastly different molecules is nothing short of confusing and muddies the conversation. The sugar found in raw fruit is the superior version called fructose. Fructose found in raw fruits is the ideal fuel for man while cooked processed sugars (removed from their natural environment of fiber, vitamins, minerals and phytonutrients and subjected to high heat) are possibly one of the most harmful things we can eat even in small quantities. The human body and all of the cells run primarily on raw fructose as the preferred fuel. Cells can use glucose also for fuel but this process requires the added step of insulin and is not the preferred fuel source. Eating too much fruit is basically impossible, the body will simply turn off the hunger mechanism upon satiation. The fact is that fructose as found in raw fruits has no resemblance to the processed sugars found in cooked desserts or breads and the idea that they behave the same way in the human body is clearly false even to the lay person.

Fruit was made to be eaten – No living creature is harmed by eating fruit. From a spiritual perspective there is no more perfect food than fruit. Fruit is the only food that was made with the specific intention that an animal is attracted to it and eats it for the purpose of spreading the seeds of the mother tree.

Should children eat fruit? – Yes! The more the better if a person wants healthy kids. Because fruit is so vital for a healthy body, it is important to encourage children to eat as much fruit as possible in their daily lives and make it easy to access. When children eat fruits as part of their regular diet they are much less likely to crave the cooked sugars in candies and sodas, which are not only destructive to the body of the child but also to their mind as demonstrated by behavioural changes in children after consuming high sugar foods or drinks.

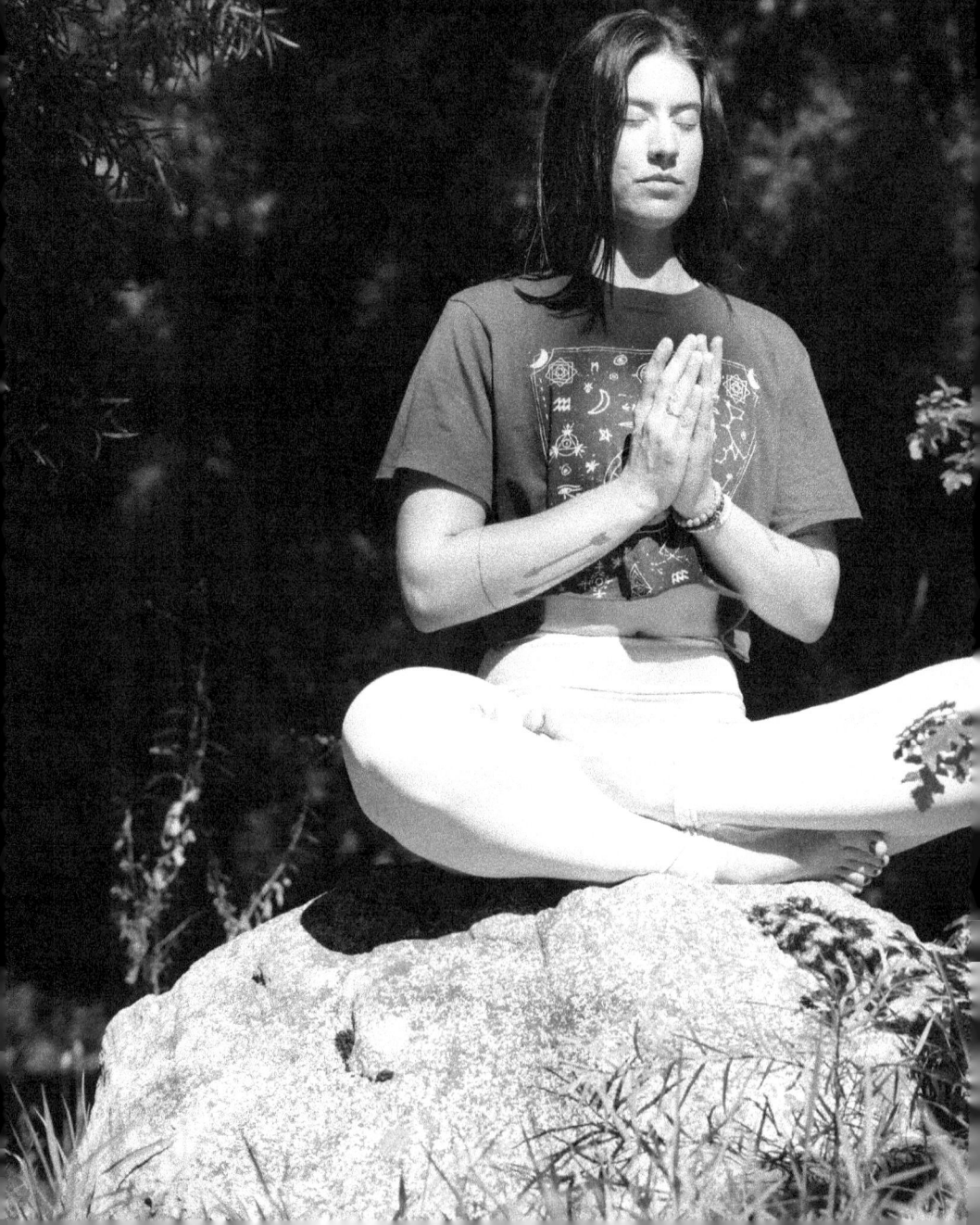

CHAPTER 19

The Mind and Subconscious

Understanding your mind and how it affects your beliefs and behaviours is not a simple endeavour, yet it is one of the most important a human can undertake. This is because our minds determine our perceptions which in turn determine our reality. While many people believe that reality is determined from outside events, the wise person realizes that reality is determined in the mind by its attitude and response to outside events.

Our mind's interpretation and experience create reality, which is ultimately completely subjective and this explains why two people can be watching the same movie and have two completely different reactions or learn completely different lessons.

Thus, given the same external environment, two different minds are capable of producing two totally different realities. Yes, beauty is indeed in the eye of the beholder, as are interpretations of reality. While standing next to each other waiting for a bus, one person will be happy and fulfilled feeling gratitude for each breath and the other completely miserable feeling like they are wasting time.

What is very important to understand is that your mind is programmed through suggestion, in other words your mind is operating based on what other people have told you. This is a key concept everyone needs to understand. Everything that you know, or think that you know, about yourself and about the world around you is the result of suggestions that have been imprinted on you since you were an infant and delivered to your subconscious mind through suggestion.

If we are aware of the power of suggestion and the effect it has on our own behaviour and way of thinking we are then able to begin the process of replacing negative, toxic suggestions with positive statements which will ideally reach our subconscious mind and result in more positive outcomes in our conscious lives.

For example, when I was a kid and would sing in the car with my sister she would always stop me mid-song and tease me saying 'you have a terrible voice'. Literally every time I would sing as a child I was told 'you have a terrible voice'. Eventually I started to believe this as fact and then I would tell myself that 'I have a terrible voice' any time there was a chance to sing in public and so I never volunteered.

Later in life I started to use my voice with chanting mantras and noticed that my voice actually was not so terrible. So now at this point in my life I have transcended the self-degrading suggestion with the new 'I have a good voice' statement which of course was the reality all along but I was suggested otherwise and believed it.

I hope this example helps you appreciate how much of what you believe about yourself to be true is simply the result of what other people told you about yourself (often for their own reasons and to serve their interests not necessarily yours). My sister was able to feel better about herself by telling me that I have a terrible voice regardless of whether it was true or not.

Suggestion imprints into the subconscious mind in the same way a vinyl record gets stamped. And, just like a vinyl record, once stamped it continues to replay the same suggestion which then dominates and informs all your present moments. Now you can see that what appears as reality to you is typically just past programs and not a true depiction of present events.

We must understand that in seeking to discover who we really are, that we must not be unduly influenced by the opinions and attitudes of others. We are all to some degree susceptible to negative suggestions that are conveyed by the people in our lives. However many such suggestions are oftentimes unfair and/or inaccurate and result in a lowered perception of oneself and one's abilities. It is very important to realize that to unlock our true potential we recognize and reprogram negativity that has entered our conscious and/or subconscious mind.

How do we accomplish this goal? The answer is through the power of meditation.

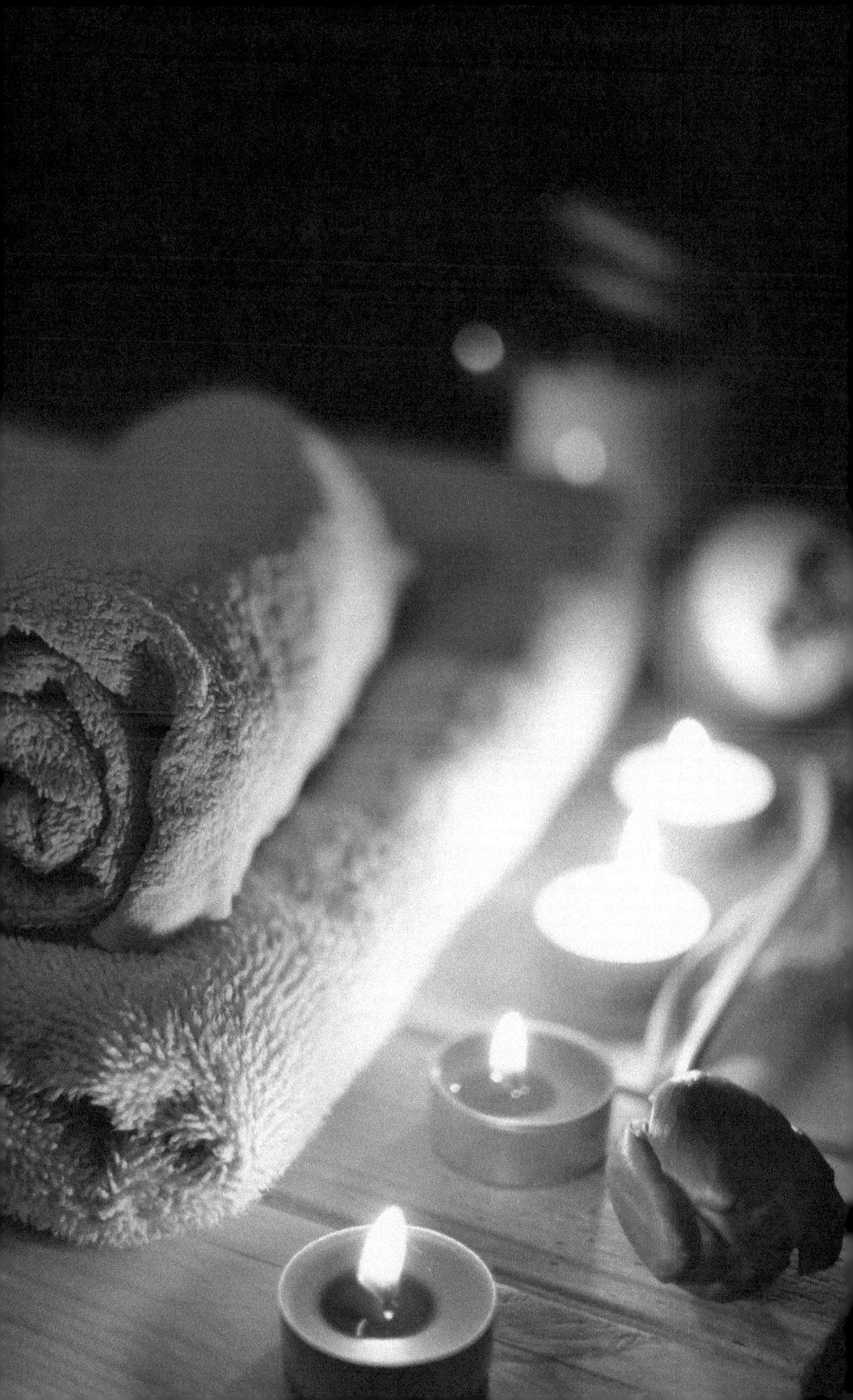

CHAPTER 20

Meditation and Reprogramming Subconscious

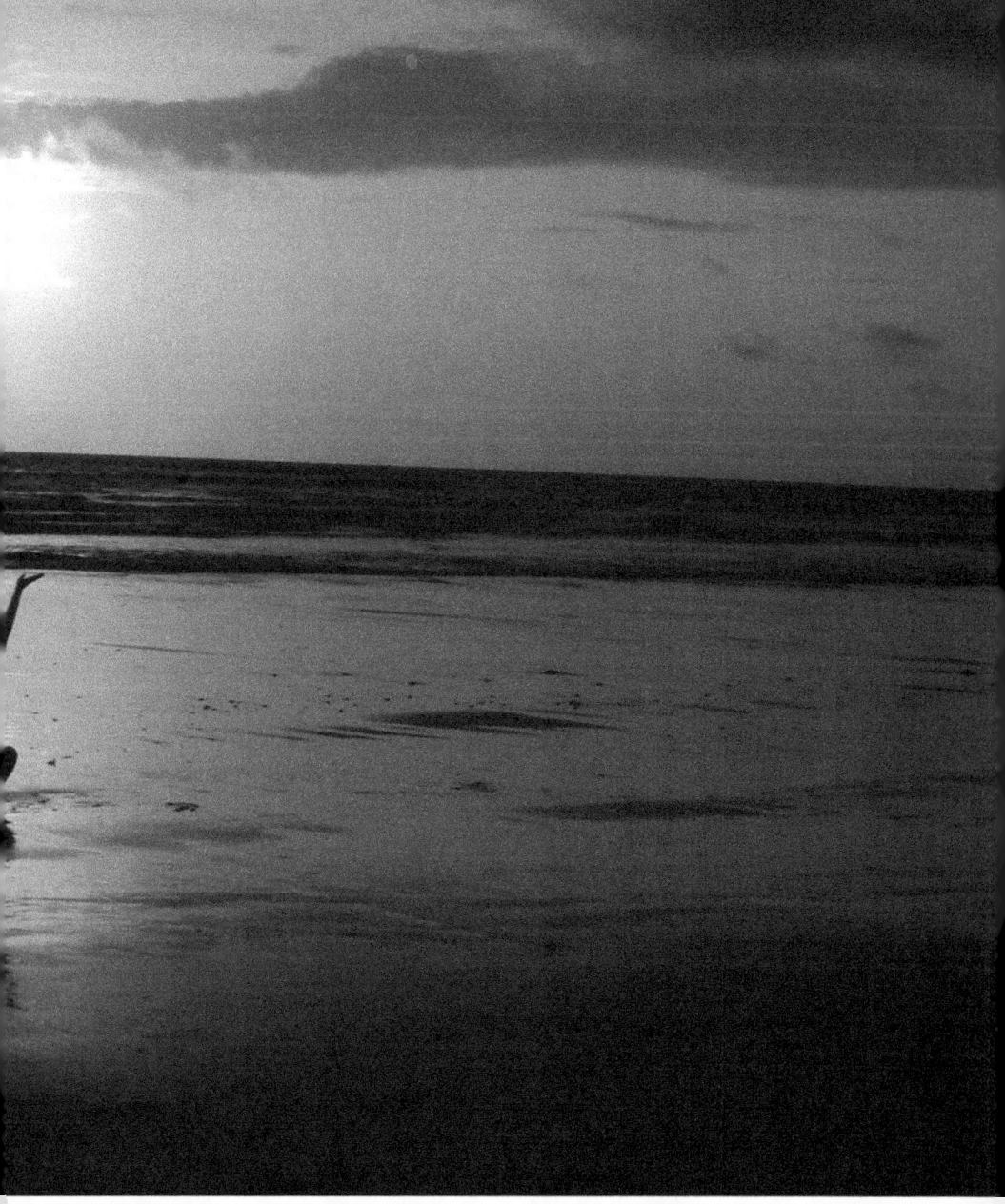

Now that it is understood how the subconscious mind gets programmed through suggestion, the next task is to learn how to use this knowledge to become healthier and more enlightened.

The subconscious mind must be presented information directly. The definition of suggestion is the direct presentation of an idea to the mind. The subconscious mind is a loyal servant and faithful absorber of all that it is presented. And, since the subconscious mind is informing all of your waking moments, this becomes a direct mechanism for controlling or influencing reality in a person.

There are many suggestions that we encounter in our everyday lives. Suggestions given to us by others are often very influential. Many things can form suggestions. Music is a suggestion. The environment is a suggestion. The lanes on a road are a suggestion. Every single advertisement that you are exposed to is suggestion.

But of all the possible avenues to communicate with our subconscious mind the most effective is the power of auto-suggestion or self-suggestion. The fact is that what we say to ourselves is the most important part of our life and can determine everything about our present and future. Our subconscious mind listens to everything we say and records it so it can reflect it back through the conscious mind's experience.

This is where meditation according to yoga comes into the equation. Meditation according to yoga involves 8 Steps known as the Ashtanga yoga system and one of these 8 Steps is Dhyana or Suggestion. In the Yoga Sutras, Patanjali explains the concept of suggestion.

Within a state of profound stillness of the body–mind there is found access to the subconscious mind programming levels. It is as if with deep meditative states the glacier of the subconscious mind emerges above the surface, allowing for new impressions to be made which replace the pre-existing or negative thought patterns.

This is why meditation is one of our keys to personal transformation and evolution. This type of meditation is not easily absorbed from books and is one of the daily classes taught at Medellin Wellness Center where this system is showcased.

CHAPTER 21

Patterns

Unconscious patterns in life are like programs that continue to play without any awareness. Resulting from previous suggestions and the fact that energy flows towards the path of least resistance, we find ourselves repeating behaviors without awareness and without regard for their results.

Many people are in fact not happy or fulfilled because they are living life through an expression of unconscious patterns and previously delivered suggestions and this creates suffering since it is all past rather than present moment.

Sometimes people gain awareness that they are doing certain habits without awareness and that these actions are having deleterious effects on their life.

At this point most people will determine that in order to improve their situation they must change their behaviors. This desire to change and the subsequent forcing of change must be very carefully managed if not transcended. Forcing a change of behaviour is not the best way because it is not sustainable and leads to other results like resentment.

One of the most important things to recognize is that we don't need to force change of behavior. Many of us waste energy trying to force behavioral change which ends up suppressing desires and creating harmful psychological damage.

The key to transformation is not forcing change but to instead shining a light on the unconscious patterns that influence and direct our behavior.

Unconscious patterns are like areas of darkness in our subconscious mind which require illumination. Shining light on the mind is called awareness and is the most important skill to have on the path to mental and physical wellbeing.

Rather than trying to force a change of behavior or thinking, it is more effective to shine awareness on the nature of the unconscious pattern which then illuminates that area and dissolves the pattern under its light. An unconscious pattern that has been illuminated by awareness is not an unconscious pattern anymore.

When we bring awareness to the context of the situation or behavior, and experience compassion towards ourselves, we fortify ourselves so that we will be stronger when we next confront the potential for repeating the pattern. This awareness and compassion combination is a powerful ally on the path of life.

Most people are so busy criticizing and judging themselves for their perceived faults that they don't have the energy to make a more aware decision next time. The attempt to force change as a result of negative self judgement leads to even more suffering.

By having awareness and then compassion and forgiveness, and surrendering to your previous actions, you bring great strength to your overall being allowing you the power and freedom to make change if you choose. This shall be explored in more detail in the following chapter.

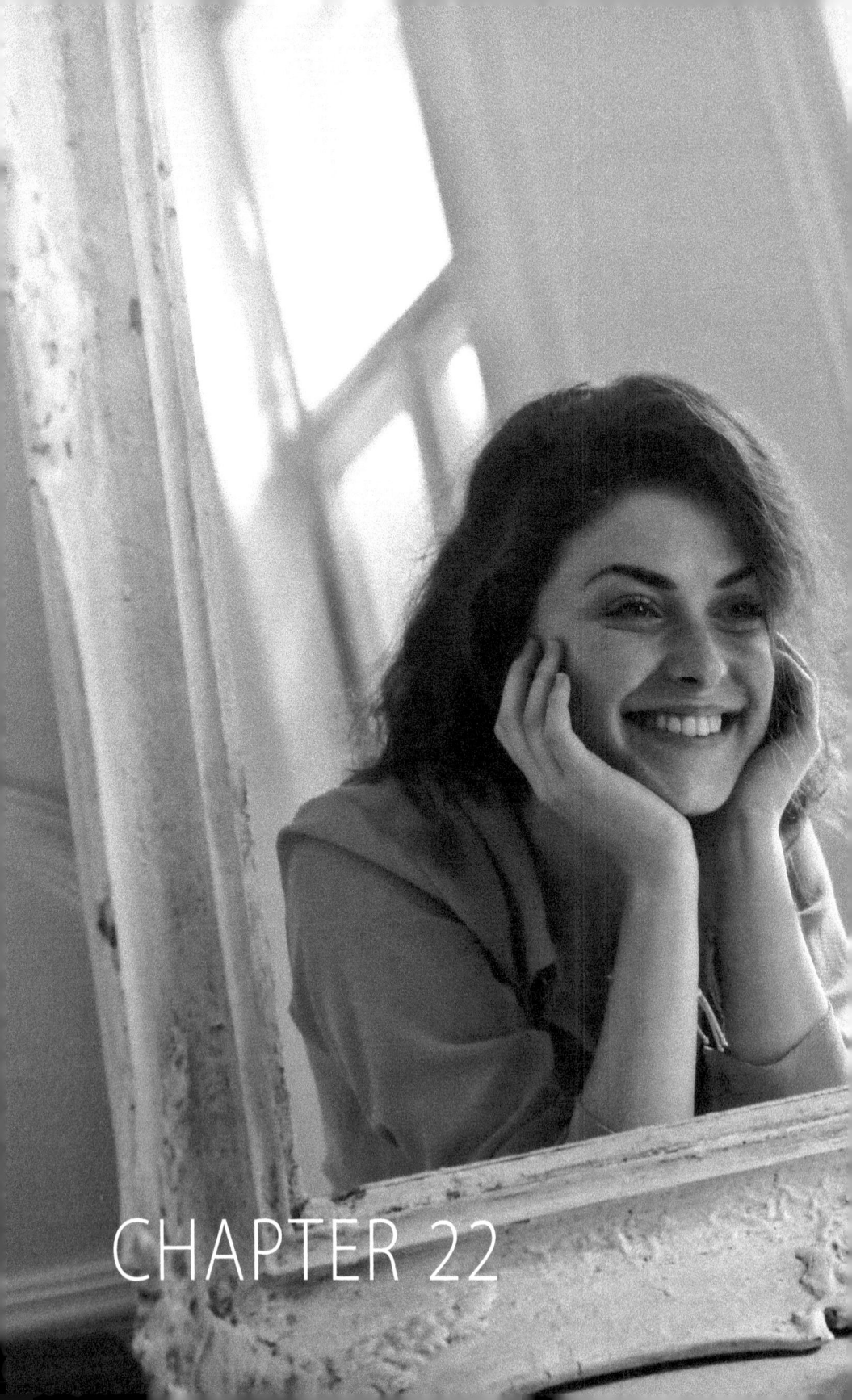

CHAPTER 22

Analysis vs Self Judgement or Criticism

Most people, upon looking at the results in front of them, seek ways to improve the quality of their lives and feel frustrated when things are not working out the way they hoped or expected. It is not uncommon for us to look back at our past mistakes and blame ourselves for the failures and disappointments we all experience. Unfortunately this can negatively and unfairly affect our level of consciousness as self-criticism is extremely destructive due to the power of suggestion discussed earlier.

Instead of self-judgement it is better to apply something called self-analysis.

Self-analysis may appear similar but is actually completely different from self-criticism and self-judgement and should not be confused. Self-analysis is a useful and important way of understanding why we behave the way we do and should be followed by a relaxed consideration of whether we wish to continue such behaviour based on the results.

Self-analysis is an open and honest process of self-evaluation that does not contain any judgement or criticism – being able to see that we have acted in a way that was not ideal without mentally punishing ourselves for being a bad person or doing wrong. The self-punishment that we inflict on ourselves is one of the most destructive forces we can unleash.

Many people are interested in self-improvement but choose to punish themselves for past mistakes in the mistaken belief that some sort of atonement is necessary for reform or improvement of future actions. Do not punish or blame yourselves for your past mistakes. We are human and errors are unavoidable and inevitable and many times beyond our conscious control. Rather, if you feel compassion for yourself and the imperfections of others, you will discover how powerful compassion is at creating harmony and peace in your lives.

By not engaging in self-punishment we are able to save a lot of energy which can then be used for a purpose more in line with our goals and intentions. In other words, when we are not punishing ourselves for our mistakes, we have energy and a positive attitude and will be more able to not repeat mistakes. This ability results in more harmony and fulfilment in our lives.

Our minds must be used for awareness and not for self-criticism. When we use our minds to shine awareness on our behavioral patterns we are able to understand their source which is often a program or suggestion or trauma that created a pain that we did not want to experience. Being aware of the source of an unconscious pattern helps to take its power away as a person can focus awareness on compassion and understanding instead of self-punishment and self-torture.

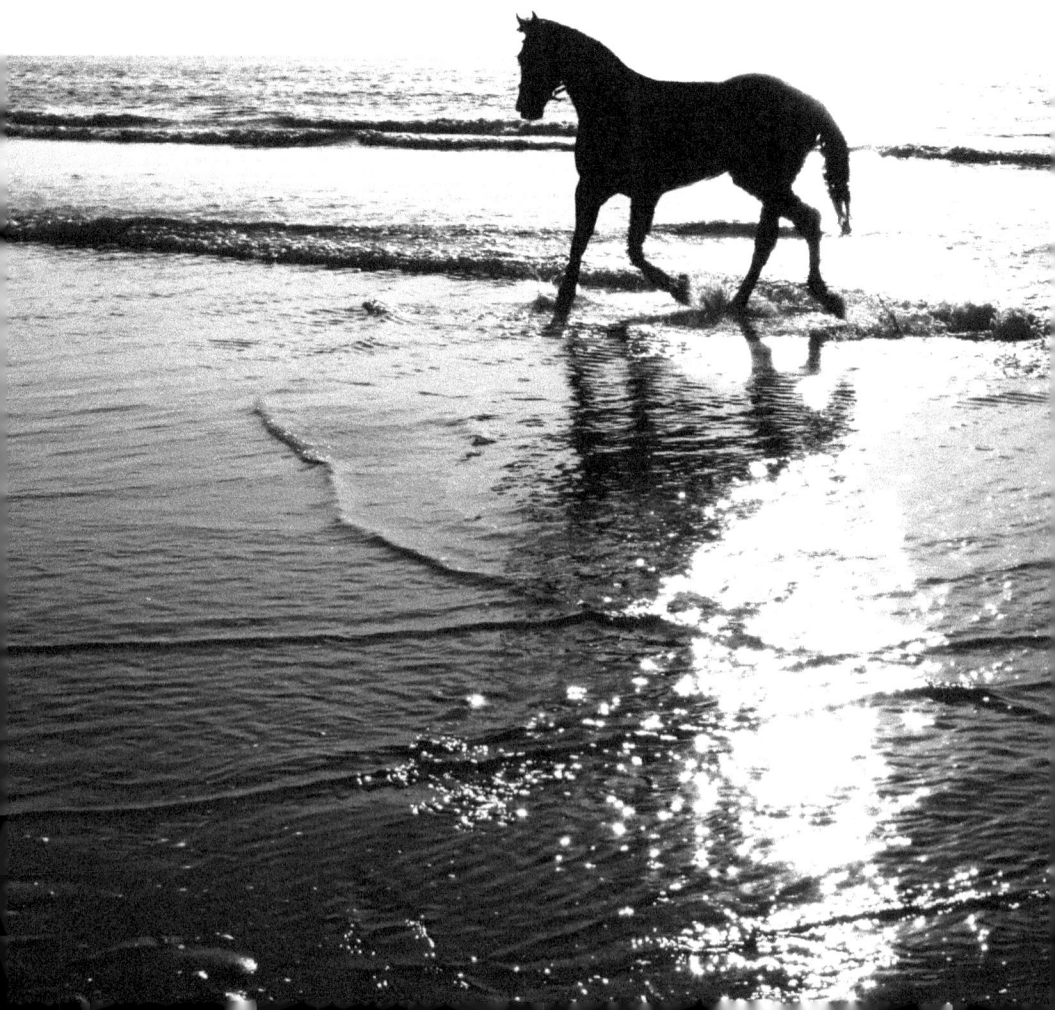

CHAPTER 23

Avoiding and Reversing Depression

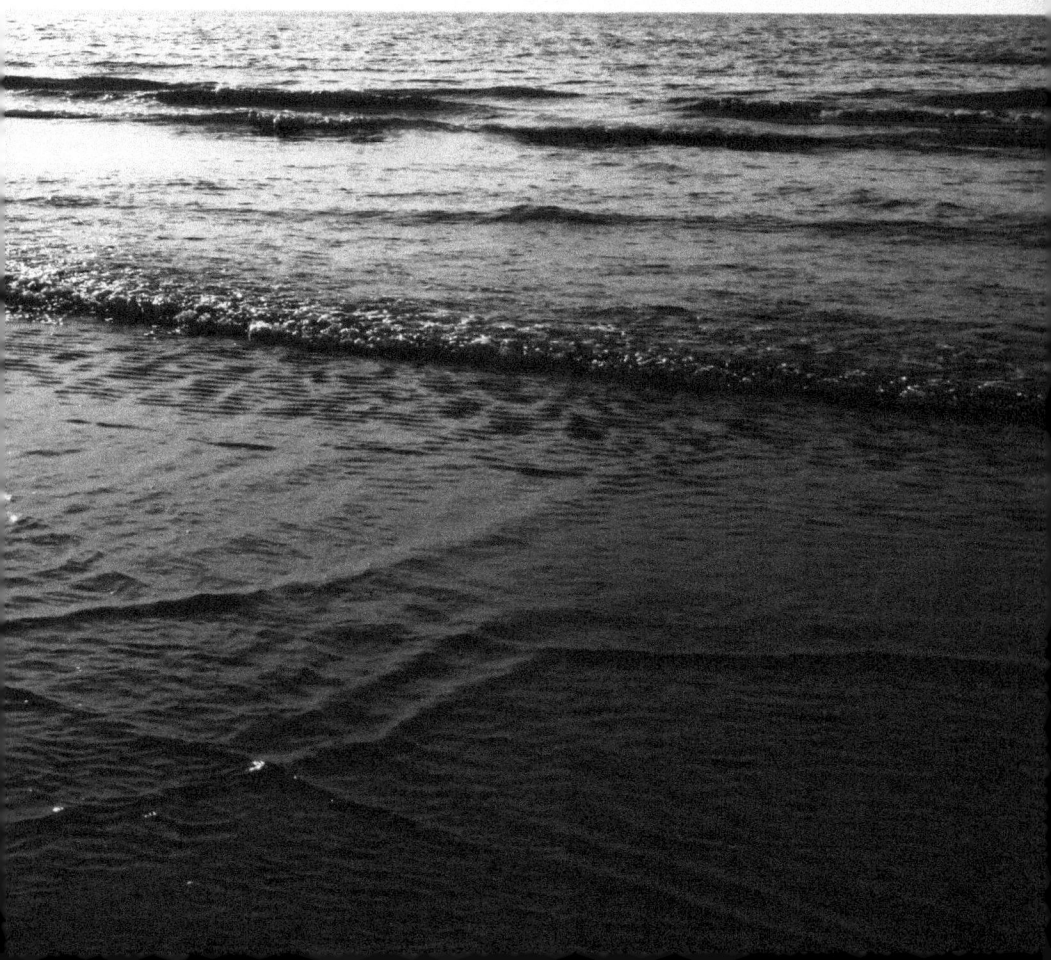

For many people, depression is a chronic and debilitating condition that can result from mental and physical illness. Unfortunately modern medicine is focused on treating depression as a medical condition which can only be effectively managed with pharmaceutical drugs while ignoring the role that an unhealthy diet, lack of exercise, and the inability to reduce stress can contribute to chronic depression.

Anybody who does not exercise every day is basically asking for depression. The point is that depression is the natural state of a mind that is attached to a degraded body system.

One of the great failures of the modern pharmaceutical approach to depression and mental imbalances is that it does not consider the pathology that is created by poor food choices, a body that is stagnated due to lack of movement, and factors like sleep deprivation or the effects of toxic exposure on the nervous system.

The mind is an organ in the body just like the heart or the lungs. And just like these other organs the brain can function in either a healthy or unhealthy way. And just as poor diet and lack of exercise negatively affect the heart and lungs so too do they affect the mind. A mind that is not functioning in health will tend towards depression and fear. This is what most people experiencing psychological symptoms are living with: an unhealthy body creating an unhealthy mind which expresses itself as depression.

Voltaire's quote is particularly apt in the context of typical treatment of mental health: 'Doctors are men who give drugs of which they know little to cure diseases of which they know less to humans of which they know nothing.'

There is no subject that medical men know less about than the human mind.

Oftentimes loneliness is associated with depression. This connection between loneliness and depression is common thus it is important to note a distinction between being alone and feeling lonely. They are not the same and just because a person is alone does not mean that they need to be lonely. Conversely, many people are lonely while surrounded by other people.

Humans are gregarious and social creatures by nature so, for many people, being alone leads to a feeling of being lonely which results in feeling stressed and depressed.

One very effective solution to this potential sense of feeling lonely or isolated is learning to practice meditation. Meditation is how we move from feeling loneliness to experiencing the peace of aloneness.

Meditation helps us to still and reprogram the mind and to understand our place in this mysterious universe. This can bring peace, harmony and a sense of belonging into our heart and mind which is also called fulfilment, which is the goal of human consciousness as opposed to some ecstatic 'happiness' that remains elusive and in any event is unsustainable.

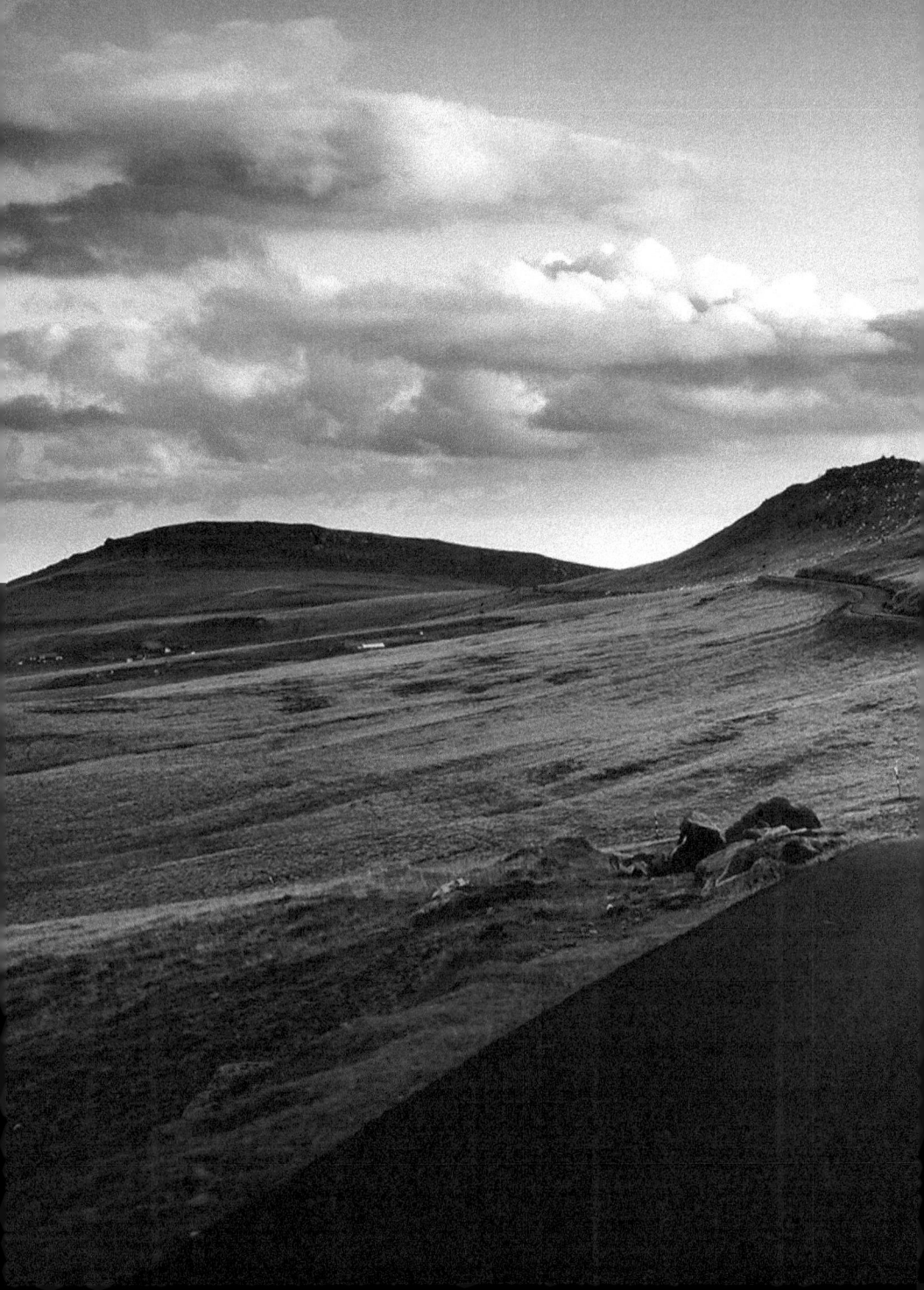

CHAPTER 24

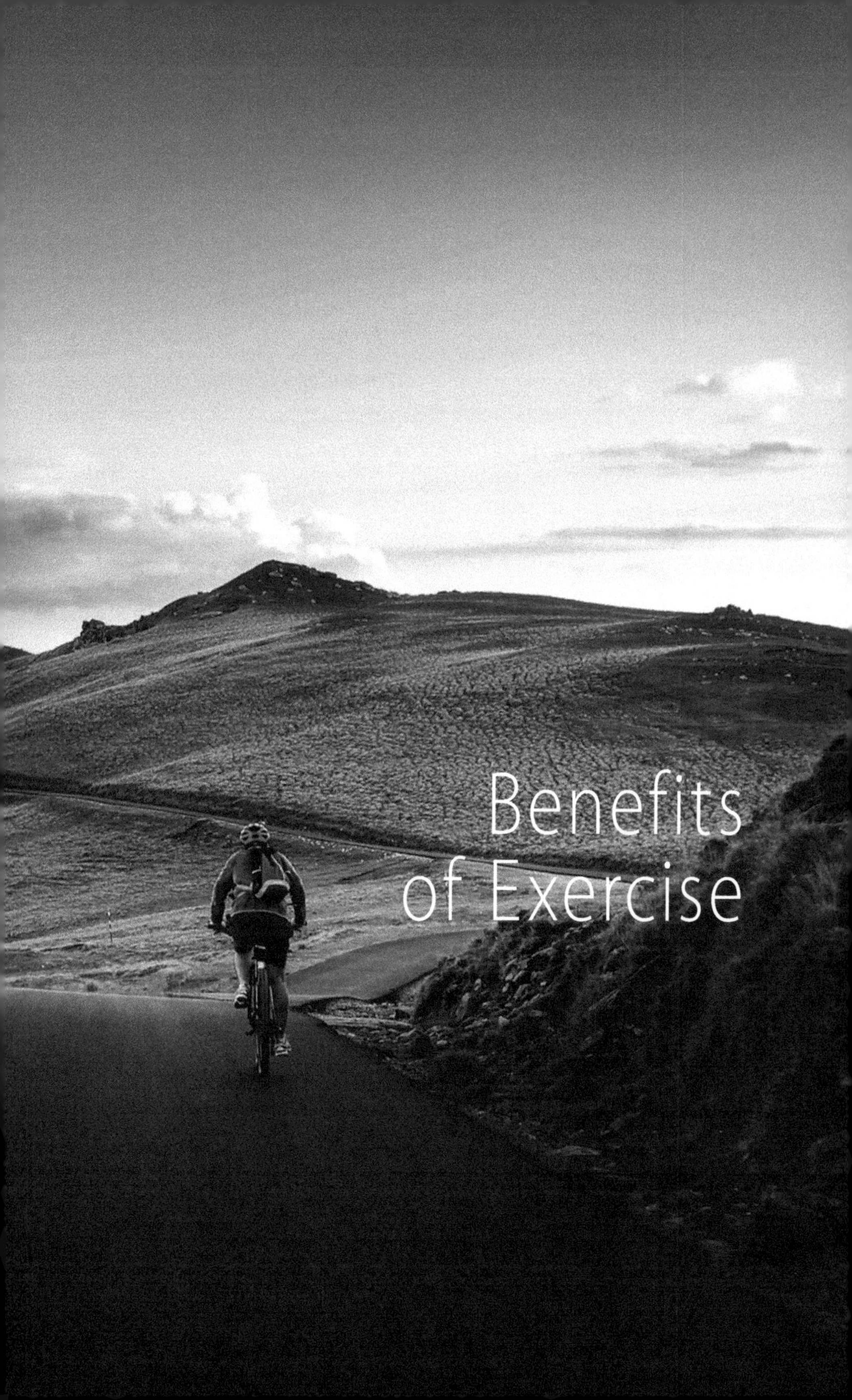

Benefits
of Exercise

Regular exercise offers protective powers that help to strengthen the immune system and prevent early degeneration and disease.

Note to readers: Those people who are relatively healthy and with good energy levels should exercise as vigorously as possible for between approximately 45 minutes to an hour each day. Those people who are not at full strength due to health conditions should exercise more moderately, engaging in walking and light movement practices.

Regular exercise will promote and result in superior health as follows:

Immune system – People who exercise regularly are healthier and more resilient than those who do not. Exercise stimulates the body's circulation of the blood and lymph allowing the immune system to operate efficiently throughout the body.

Mind – A mind, which is a physical organ of the body, attached to a body that does not exercise is not likely a healthy mind. It is very difficult to have a healthy mind without a healthy body. A body that does not exercise will create a mind that feels anxious and nervous. When there is too much nervous energy in the system and it is not released positively through exercise it gets directed back into the system and expresses itself as stress.

Circulation – Blood flow is what carries oxygen and nutrients through the body and when we exercise blood is flowing faster and under greater pressure which means oxygen and nutrients are being delivered to the deeper regions. A sedentary lifestyle results in impaired circulation and is directly related to the development of conditions including edema (swelling) and blood clots, to name just a few. The human body thrives on movement and activity which promotes proper circulation throughout the body. The body was made for activity and the circulation of the fluids of the body is based on movement-based physics. This is why a modern quote says 'sitting is the new smoking'.

Lymphatic – The lymphatic system houses the body's immune system and is also responsible for the removal of waste. In the same way that we would not want our sewage pipes and drainage lines to not have insufficient circulation and flow as this would create stagnation, lack of exercise creates stagnation of the lymph which can lead to acid buildup and degenerative disease conditions. Regular exercise is the mechanical means the body uses to circulate its fluids and energy.

Muscular – Despite popular belief, strong muscles do not come from eating protein. Nobody can eat themselves to strength. Only exercise can create and maintain muscular strength and as the old saying goes 'you either use it or lose it'. Muscles are living cells that respond to stress and when asked to overcome challenging circumstances they respond by growing and getting bigger or maintaining their size. Anybody who has ever experienced an illness or injury that requires prolonged bed rest is aware that muscles atrophy quickly when no longer used.

Bone density – Just like muscles, bone operates on a 'use it or lose it' basis; lack of exercise and a sedentary lifestyle will result in loss of bone density or osteoporosis. When we stop demanding our bones resist our weight and stop putting stress on the bones through exercise or other activity, the bones will naturally lose their density. It is not a function of aging as many wish to believe but rather a function of time passing without demanding anything from the bones. Osteoporosis is not

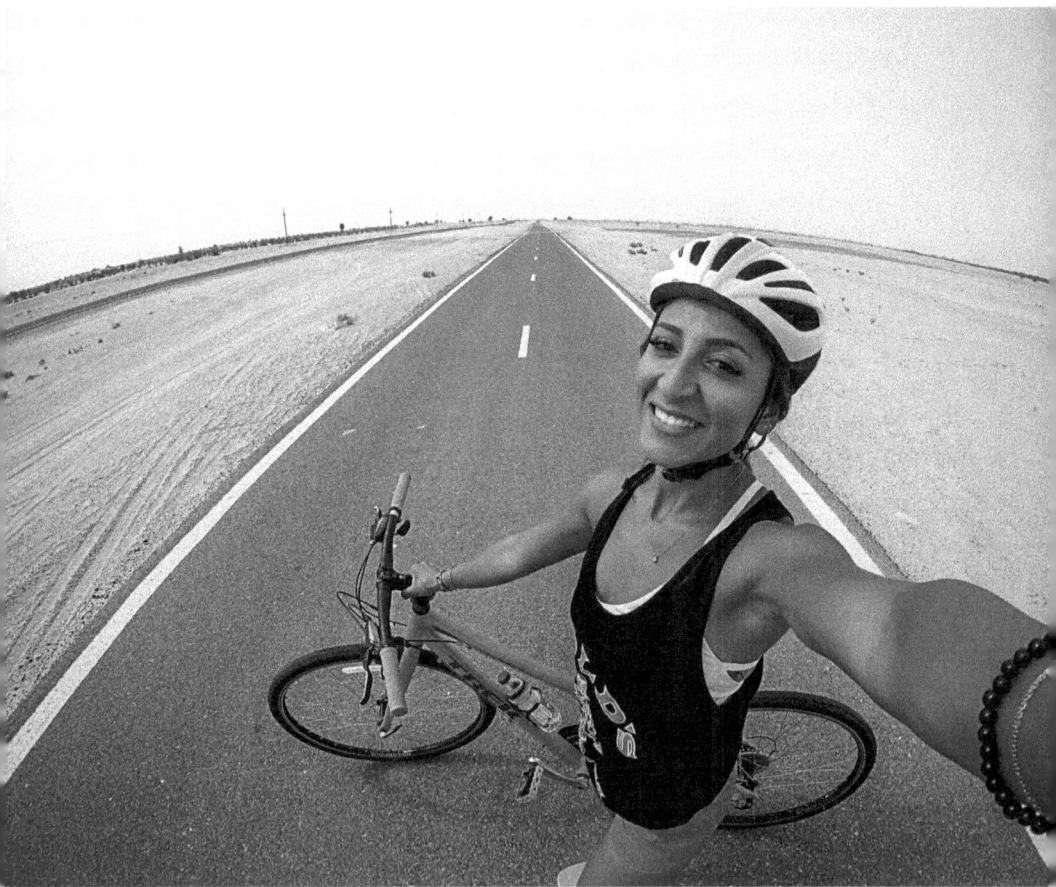

caused by a lack of dairy in the diet. Calcium from dairy is not used as the dairy industry wishes us to believe. The body does not use the calcium found in milk because it is too busy trying to neutralize the acidic effect on the blood that dairy produces, using its alkaline minerals like calcium to do so. Osteoporosis is not found in cultures where adults do not consume dairy.

Make it a lifestyle – Exercise must be a lifestyle and enjoyable because it is easier to commit to something every day that you enjoy than something that you resist or feel is a punishment or a requirement. One way to enjoy exercise is to feel intense gratitude for having a physical body to exercise. Many people live in bodies that are unable to do many different types of exercise and being able to walk or do yoga or swim or bike is a great blessing and this must remain at the forefront of your attitude. Yoga in particular is great because most people enjoy it and, when properly applied, it can provide the body with the optimal benefit of exercise.

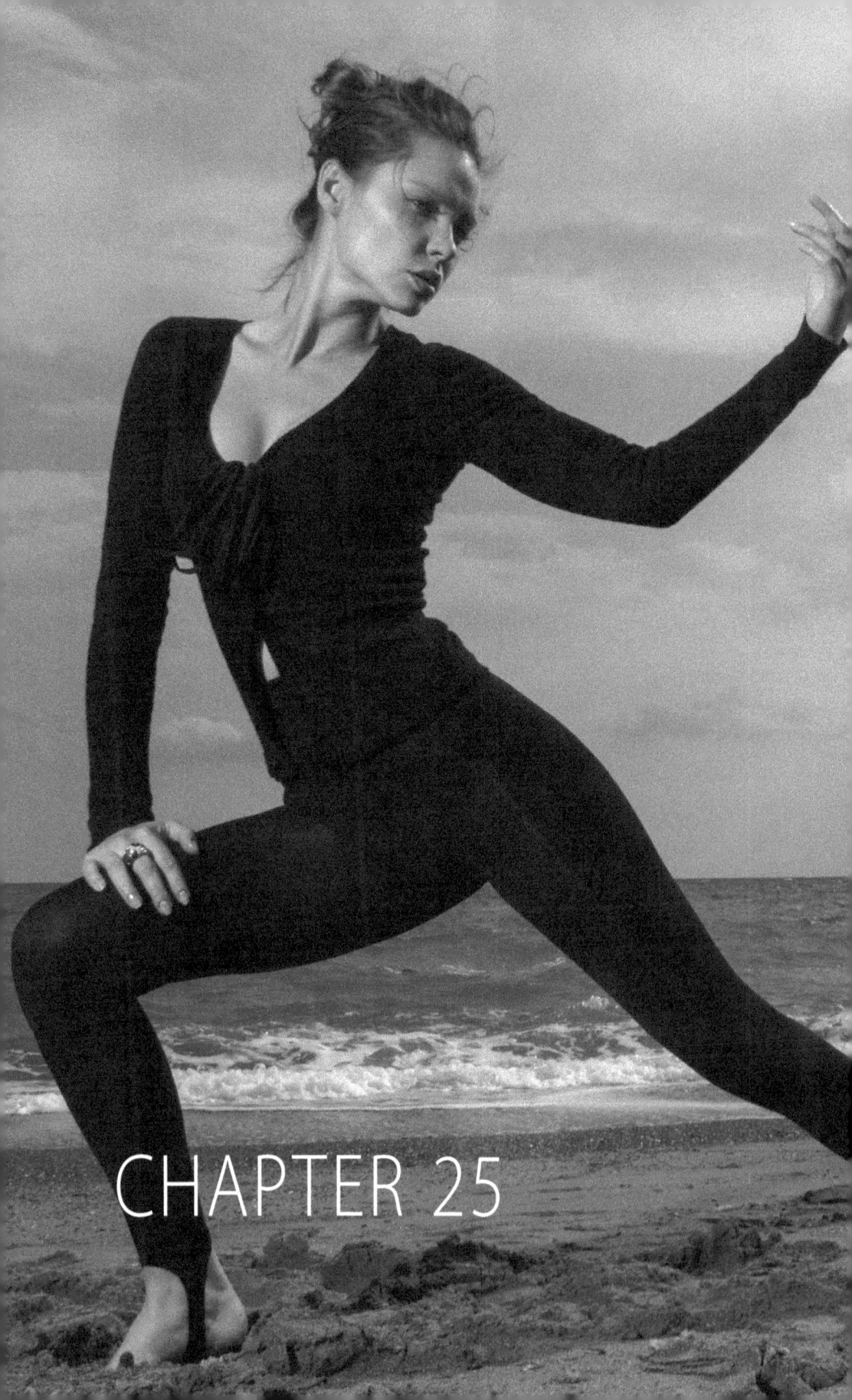

CHAPTER 25

Daily Exercise
Is Best

The best approach to exercise is *'no days off...no exceptions'*. This approach is best for many reasons, not the least of which is that it precludes thinking about it. The only question of your day becomes *when* you are going to exercise not *if*.

Humans like all animals must exercise their body every single day because that is how we are designed by nature. Do you know of any animals in nature that take a day off from being themselves or moving in their natural way?

As mentioned earlier, proper circulation is literally dependent on movement of the body. While most people visualize that the heart itself is pumping the blood all around the body this is not the case completely. The circulatory system relies on muscular contraction to move blood up the venous vessels back to the heart.

The heart only really efficiently pumps the blood to the capillaries. From the capillaries it is the action of *muscular contraction* in concert with the one-way valve system that veins have that are more responsible for pushing blood back to the heart than the heart itself. Exercise therefore is literally the other half of the circulatory system.

So, it can be said that a day off from exercise is essentially a day off from efficiently circulating your blood properly around the body. These fluids bring the life energy and remove the waste matter from the system which keeps it functioning well.

For most of us the best time to exercise is the very first thing in the morning, even before breakfast.

Most highly successful people have a discipline that involves a morning exercise regimen. Morning exercise sets the tone for the day and allows you to enjoy the benefits of having exercised for the whole day.

MORNING EXERCISE OFFERS THE FOLLOWING BENEFITS:

When a person practices a discipline or exercises first thing in the morning the day's events cannot interfere with intention to exercise. We are all aware of how sometimes the day can get out of our control, especially if we have a family to manage, and then the exercise gets sacrificed for that day. As such, it is a very good idea to practice or exercise first thing in the morning so that it will always get done!

Morning exercise is best done on an empty stomach although fruit smoothies or fruit before exercise is always ok because fruit digests in 10 minutes and the stomach is not loaded down with work.

Practicing in the morning means we will have full energy. Exercise is always best when we are feeling energized. To exercise after working when we are tired is not ideal but night-time exercise is certainly better than no exercise at all. In cases of evening exhaustion, it is advisable to take a short rest before exercise.

The bottom line is exercising each and every day is a key component to success in strengthening the immune system and to the overall health of body and mind.

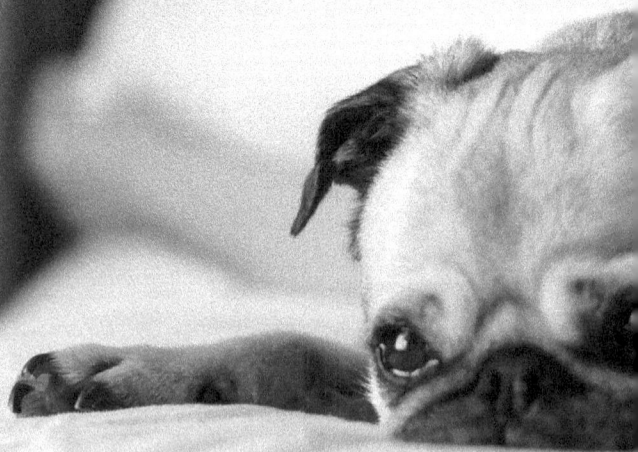

CHAPTER 26

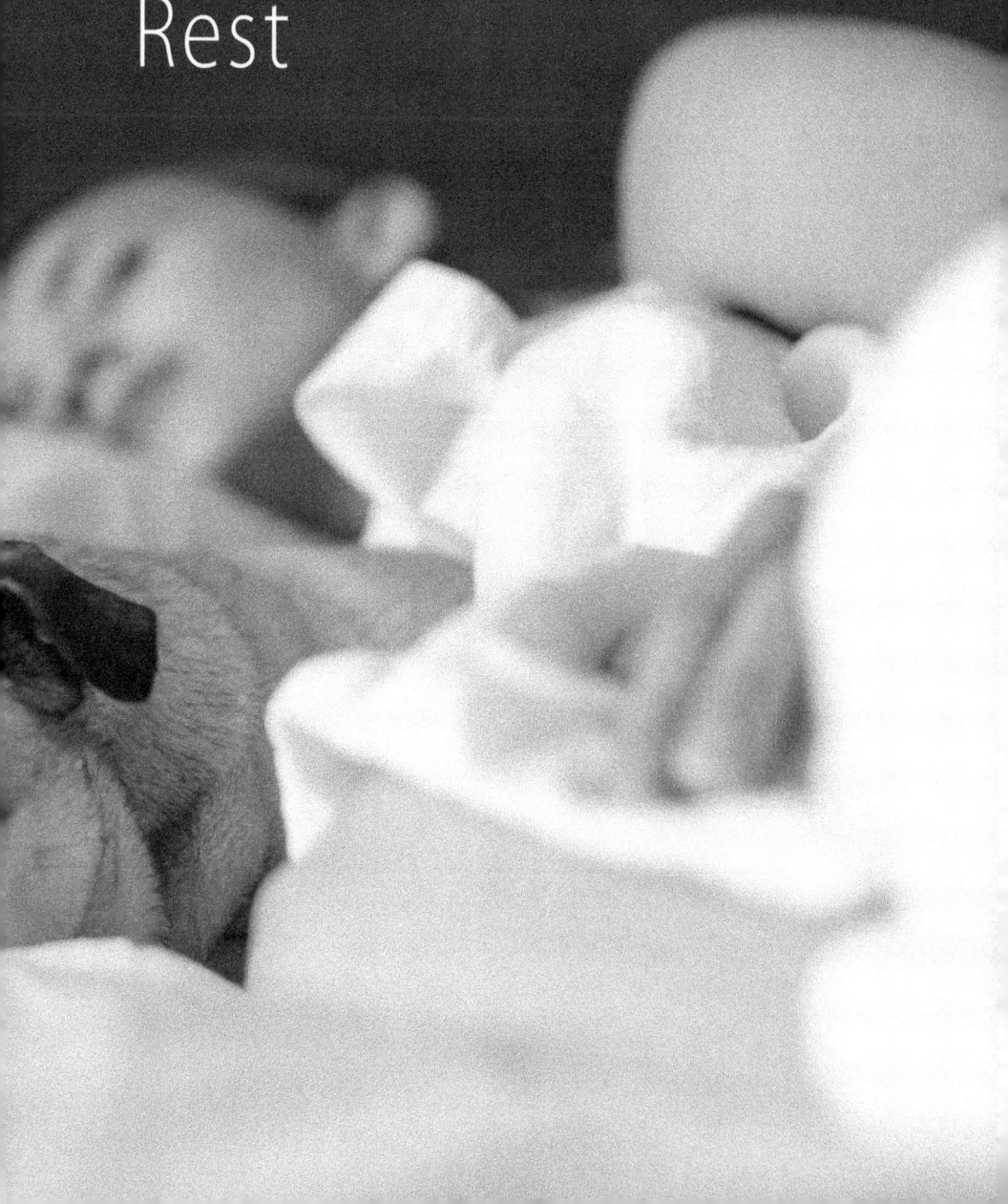

Rest

One of the most important and often overlooked of the Five Fundamental Factors is Rest.

In today's complicated and stressful world, sleep deprivation is a major health issue.

Lack of sleep creates a stressful environment in the body. Sleep deprivation has a debilitating effect on your body similar to alcohol consumption and adversely affects all dimensions of a person's functioning. Sleep deprivation also rivals alcohol in its capacity to suppress the immune system. If a person wanted to get sick the very best way to accomplish the goal would be to stop sleeping.

Rest and sleep provide an almost magical capacity to our body to heal itself. All healing happens during sleep which is why a person 'wakes up in the morning' feeling better when they are going through symptoms.

All rest is good but sleep is best for healing. This is why short or even long naps are highly prized for healing and for immune system strength overall.

Rest can take different forms and all are valuable in their own right because of the relationship between relaxation and the healing process.

Rest, relaxation and healing are highly related. One cannot have healing without relaxation and cannot have rest and relaxation that is not healing. They are essentially the same experience and function into and through the parasympathetic nervous system. When the mind feels a sense of relaxation, the body shifts to healing mode. The state of relaxation experienced in sleep and rest activates the forces of the parasympathetic nervous system which translates directly to healing capacity.

During restful sleep the body recovers and heals. Everybody has experience of waking up in the morning and feeling better than the night before. A good night of sleep is a magic healing elixir. Good sleep also keeps us looking younger and sleep has been called 'nature's cosmetic'.

Sleep is especially restorative of the nervous system. The brain is an electricity generating and transmitting organ that uses about 12 times the energy of the physical muscles. Anybody who has worked at a desk or spent long hours reading are familiar with feeling physical and mental exhaustion that seems almost insurmountable.

When people experience this fatigue many will turn to stimulants like coffee and sugar. This creates a short term surge of artificial energy as the adrenal glands are stressed and squeezed and followed by a deeper level of exhaustion which only another cup of coffee or a chocolate candy can overcome. This is a deeply unhealthy cycle which can be avoided by resting and eating more fruits at the desk.

Paradoxically drugging ourselves to stay energetic during the day oftentimes causes insomnia at night. This is because instead of listening to our bodies' need for a short rest we stimulate the body and innervate the nervous system so that it is chronically wired and overcharged. A nervous system so stimulated is unable to relax normally at night when it is time to rest, requiring in many people the unfortunate need to take a pill to sleep at night.

Let's now explore some specifics for making sure you are getting the rest your body needs:

Go to sleep early enough – If your work or school schedule requires you to wake up early in the morning the best solution is to go to sleep at an hour that will provide you with adequate restorative sleep.

What is enough sleep? The *average* adult needs between 6 – 8 hours, with some minimal variation. If you don't get the amount of sleep your body needs this will, with certainty, result in harmful sleep deprivation effects. One notable exception is when we are detoxifying or engaging in a healing event when we may require much more sleep for short periods of time while the body does extraordinary work

How do you know you got enough sleep? A person who is well rested will wake up on their own without any need for external alarm and will also wake up feeling refreshed and without the need for a morning coffee. Restorative sleep is critical to staying healthy not just physically but mentally.

The mind especially does not function well with lack of sleep as most of us know from experience. Here are a few ways of recovering your nervous energy during the day:

Nap or siesta instead of lunch – Eating can be done at the desk by snacking on fruits or drinking smoothies during the workday. However there is not a better time during the day than your lunch break to take a good rest or nap so use that time wisely.

In certain Asian countries they have created 'sleeping pods' for office workers who are working themselves to death. But to a lesser extreme in the US and Europe we are working ourselves to a slower death by not resting when we can.

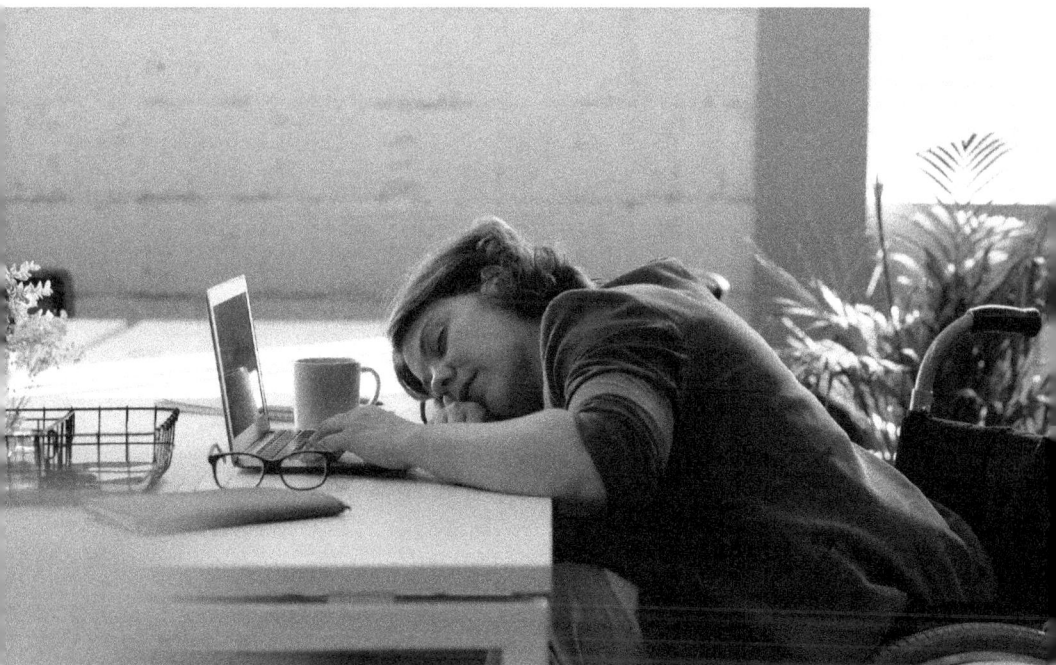

Sleep at your desk / nod off – It is likely that your boss would not like this advice on the surface but on further examination may be fully in support. And, if you are the boss then this technique can certainly work. Just allow yourself to fall asleep spontaneously at your desk for 5 or 10 minutes...even 2 minutes of sleep offers a disproportionate value to recharge the nervous system and remove fatigue.

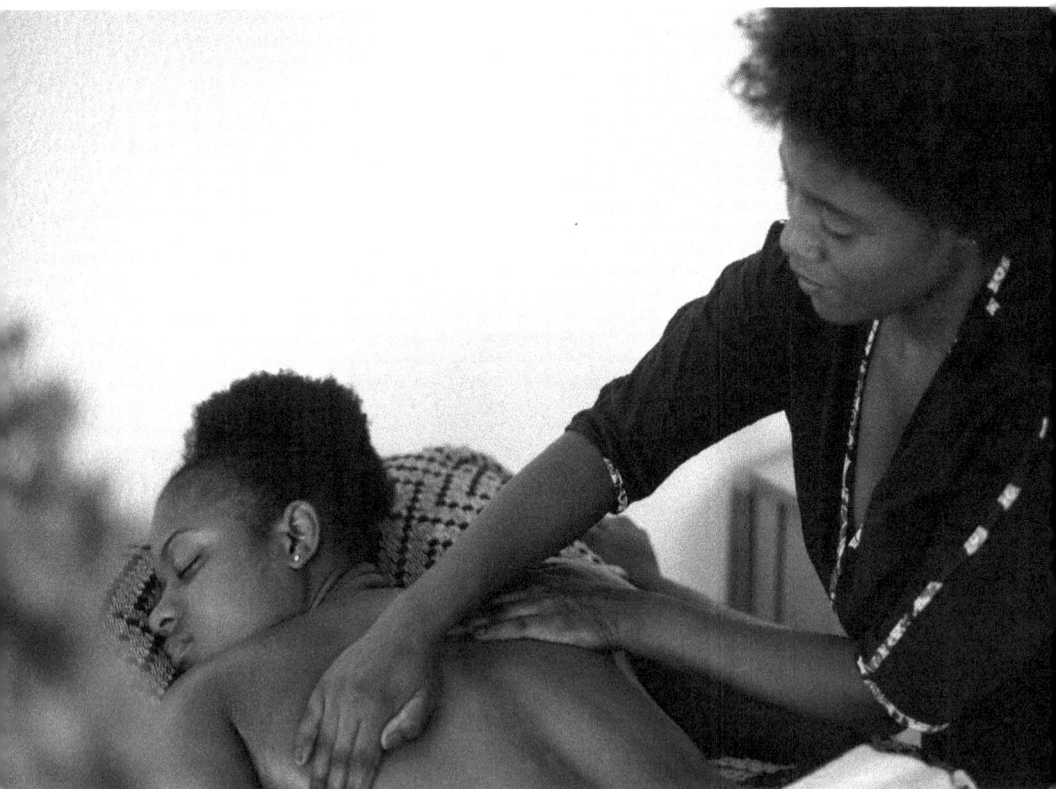

Breathe better and deeper – In addition to sleeping well, deep breathing techniques can also increase energy and promote a sense of wellbeing. Deep breathing oxygenates the body thoroughly. The breath not only delivers oxygen but also delivers a very subtle energy known in India as 'prana' and China as 'chi'. One of the unfortunate tendencies of modern man is an inability to breathe deeply and thus people live chronically low in energy for this reason as well as lack of sleep. One major benefit of exercise is that it encourages stronger and deeper breathing which oxygenates the body more thoroughly.

Guided relaxation – Because many of us find it difficult to reach a state of relaxation on our own, a guided relaxation or meditation can help people who would otherwise not be able to attain that state. Most people benefit from being guided in relaxation or meditation as it allows the subconscious mind to be suggested to all while the conscious mind is at rest.

Massage – Massage is a very effective way to relax because the healing effect of touch is profound. Sometimes only during a massage do people give themselves permission to relax. Human to human touch offers a direct way to relax a person's nervous system.

Acupuncture/acupressure – Acupuncture/acupressure is another extremely relaxing experience that also has positive energetic effects. With acupuncture the client is induced into a deep state of relaxation while needles are placed along energy meridians. With acupressure the fingers are used instead of needles. These therapeutic techniques help stimulate energy in the body to move in certain directions and the deep relaxation of the session triggers the parasympathetic nervous system which does the real deep healing work.

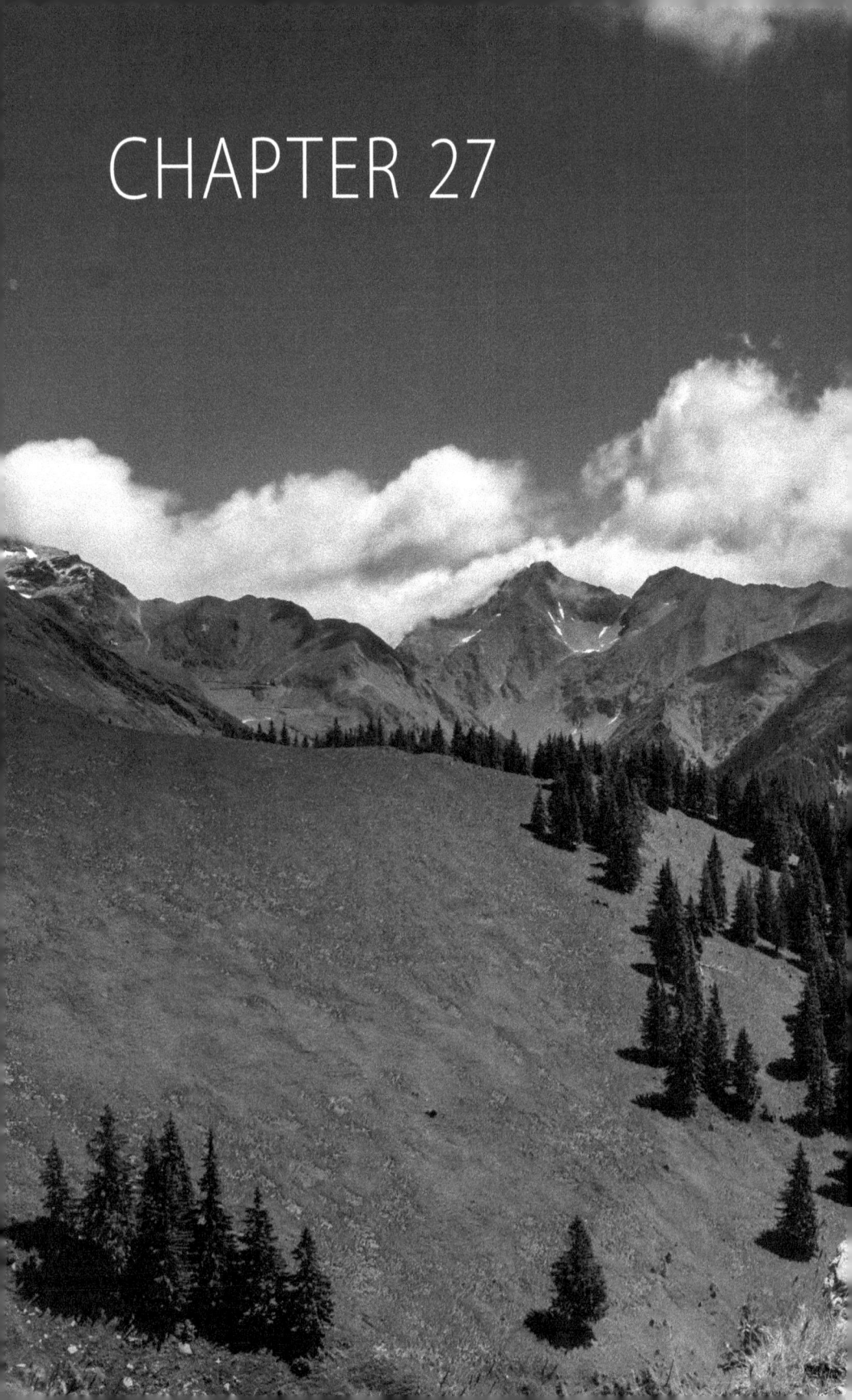

CHAPTER 27

Exercise Options

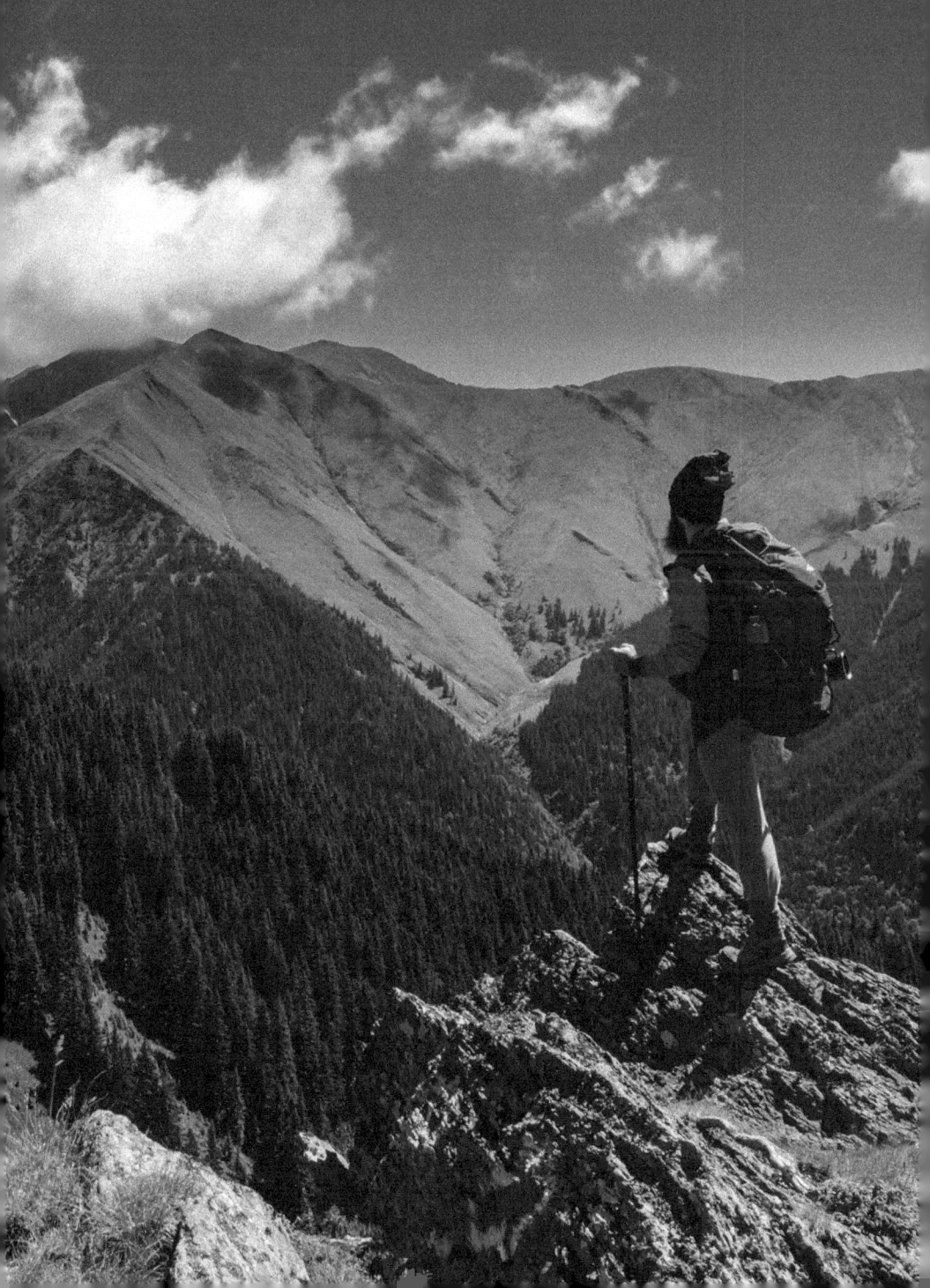

Firstly all safely performed exercise is good. Any activity that we enjoy that gets us moving around and off the couch or chair is very valuable. Every sport or physical activity that involves movement is going to be helpful to your overall wellness. That being said, some forms of exercises and practices may be more valuable than others.

If what you love to do is not on this list do not stop doing what you love unless you have a good reason. There is no need to limit yourself to only one exercise or physical activity and the below options can be a good supplement and support to your sport of choice. If you enjoy a certain sport for example there is no reason to give up playing what you love, rather the suggestion would be to add a daily practice of yoga to your regimen. See how your life improves as well as your performance whether you are an athlete or a martial artist.

For most of us, the time dedicated to exercise is limited so try to get as *much bang for your buck* as you can from your daily exercise routine by choosing one or more of the following options.

Rebounding – Rebounding is a trampoline-based exercise system that uses the principle of cellular oxygenation that results from the bouncing pulsation provided by the rebounder. Rebounding offers a benefit that is of the same quality as any cardiovascular exercise. From weight loss to bone density to overall wellbeing the rebounder is demonstrating great effectiveness in improving the immune system and overall wellbeing.

Yoga – Almost all of the wide variety of yoga styles offer many physiological benefits, such as increased muscular strength, bone density, flexibility, improved circulation, and immune/lymphatic system improvement. In addition, yoga can be a moving meditation with all the additional benefits of experiencing a one-pointed and present mind.

Swimming – This is one of the best options for exercise. Swimming provides a unique combination of cardiovascular demand with non-impact based exercise. Swimming, like yoga, is a very complete exercise system that develops a strong and resilient physical body and strong cardiovascular system.

Walking in nature – Walking in nature offers the chance to improve physical health while also connecting to nature which is in many ways a spiritual experience. Walking in Nature helps us clear our minds and see the beauty and power of the natural world and this is beneficial to the human nervous system, encouraging relaxation. Humans, like all natural creatures, do not respond well to prolonged periods without access to nature, sunshine and fresh air. Sunshine and fresh air are like nutrients that the body literally cannot live without.

Although the above referenced exercises are extremely beneficial, that fact is that **any** form of regular exercise that gets you off the couch is much better than doing nothing. So if you want to maintain good health and a sense of wellbeing, get moving!

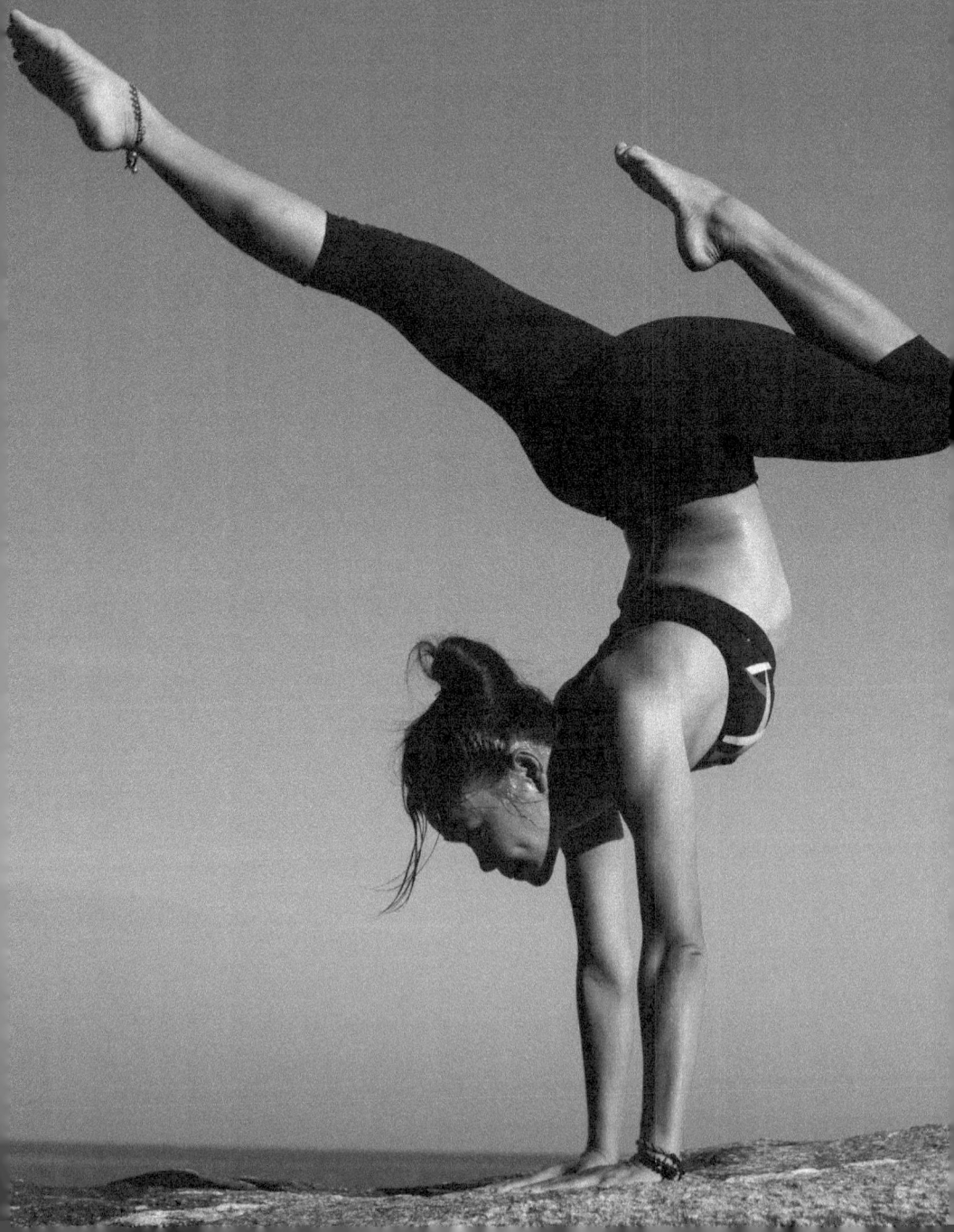

CHAPTER 28

Different Types of Yoga

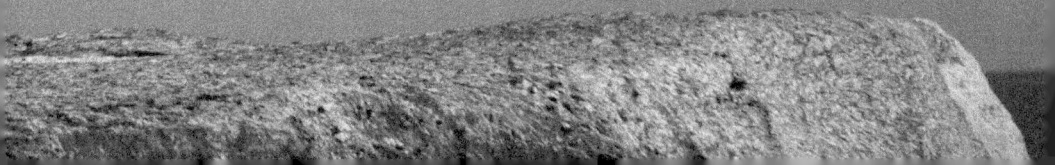

Yoga is a generic term which includes many different types of practices or paths. Yoga is both an experience and the practices designed to bring you to that experience. The experience of yoga is about identifying with eternal nature rather than our physical bodies or personalities which are always changing. Most yogis incorporate several of these paths into their sadhana (daily practices) in order to achieve the state of yoga. So again yoga is both a state of awareness as well as the practices designed to help us attain that state.

Meditation-based yoga – While most people visualize yoga as people doing different poses and breathing exercises, the deepest yoga practices are meditation based. Whether we are talking about the classical yoga of Patanjali's Yoga Sutras, Tantra, or Buddhism, the essential practice is meditation.

With some minor differences these traditions all teach meditation as a guide towards self-awareness and enlightenment. Yoga meditation reveals the unchanging and omnipresent reality behind the relatively illusory world of material and appearance.

Athletic-based yoga – Some styles of yoga direct a lot of attention to the physical benefits of practicing long flowing choreographies of yoga poses known as sequences. By practicing a comprehensive range of different asanas and obtaining a cardiovascular benefit from the flowing nature of the practice, students often experience major health benefits and a much higher quality of life. Ashtanga Vinyasa, Power Yoga, Vinyasa Yoga, and Hot Yoga are examples of athletic-based yoga. Unfortunately some yoga teachers have overemphasized the role of physical poses and this misunderstanding has led teachers to push students beyond their physical capabilities. This pushing of students who are

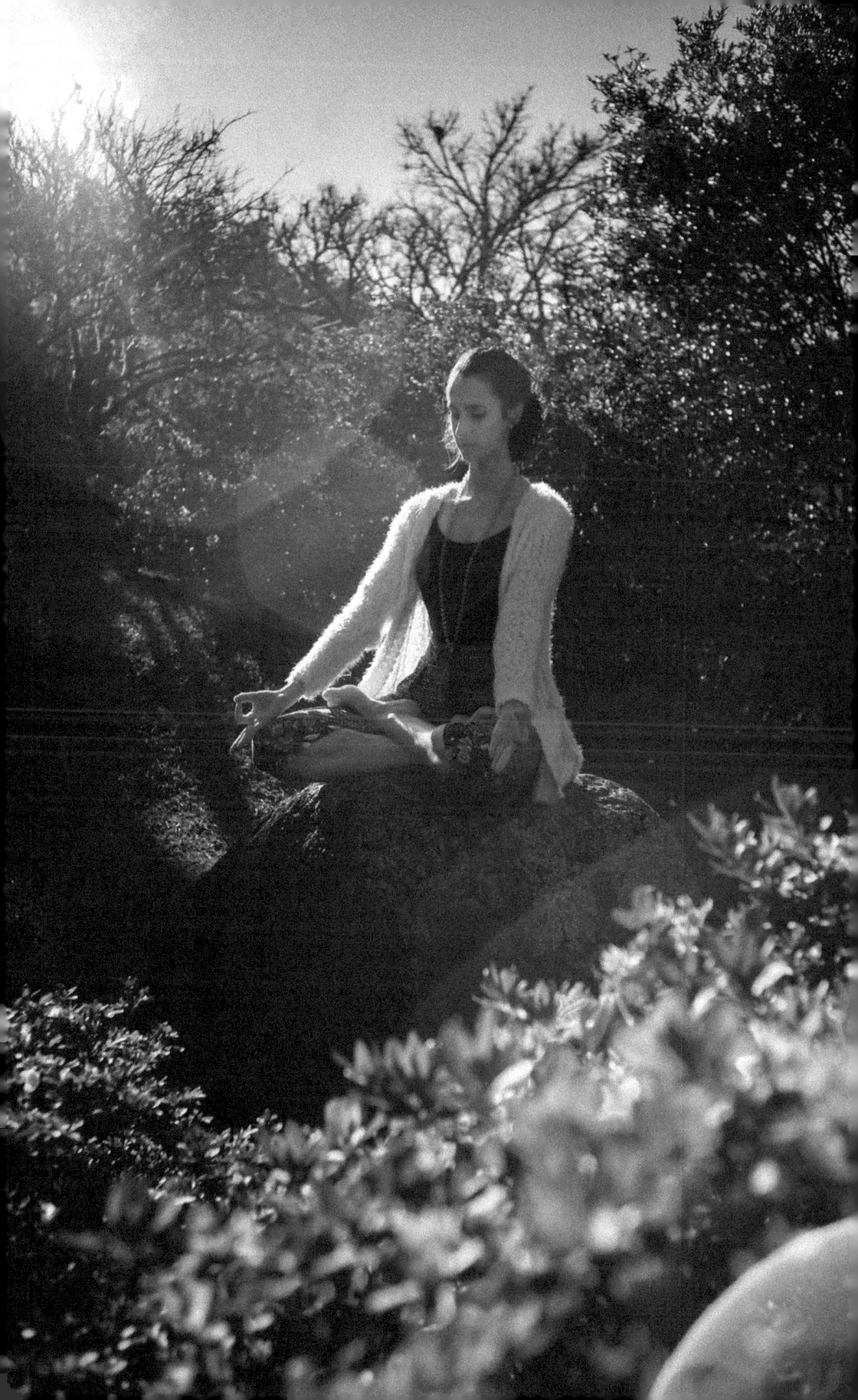

not ready commonly results in serious injuries under the false notion that advanced gymnastic performance in yoga equals advanced yoga. For this reason, these styles are best practiced with properly trained and mindful teachers who understand their student's physical abilities and limitations and always keep their best interest at heart.

Relaxation-based yoga – Some styles of yoga like Yin Yoga or Restorative Yoga are designed to help restore the energy of the student. This very valuable intention is accomplished by allowing the student to experience yoga poses while in a state of deep relaxation and while being completely supported by blankets and other props. These styles of yoga offer a profound relaxation and healing environment as rest is infused with the benefit of yoga asanas. This is valuable for all people.

Traditional Hatha Yoga – Yogis and traditions that teach Hatha Yoga as it has been taught in India over the centuries are teaching what we call in the west *Traditional Hatha Yoga*. Traditional Hatha Yoga practices involve all of the techniques students have practiced or have heard of like Asana, Pranayama, Bandha, Mudra, Mantra, Visualization and Meditation. This traditional style is not always choreographed to move with the breath but, under the guidance of an accomplished master, is more powerful than simple athletic-based practices.

Working yoga – Those people who see spirituality as an opportunity and responsibility to make the world a better place are called Karma Yogis who ask themselves how their lives can be used in the highest way to serve the will of the Divine to reduce suffering on the planet. Karma Yoga is the understanding of the truth that, if things are going to improve on earth, then we must be responsible to take action to accomplish that goal. Karma Yogis are those people who humbly and with gratitude serve humanity without asking for any type of reward or recompense.

Vibration-based yoga – The Universe ultimately is vibration and the practice that helps us resonate with that is called Nada Yoga and is perhaps the very deepest and most transformational path for those who can access it. This path suggests that by tuning into the inner sound vibration that is constantly humming within us we are able to transform our consciousness. Nada Yoga is the science of being attuned to the vibrational sound of AUM or OM. As we are vibrational beings living in a universe of magnetism and energy, when we are able to concentrate on the inner sound it is similar to receiving a cosmic download.

As mentioned earlier in the chapter, yoga practices have many distinctions as well as many common threads, however it is important to understand that these all strive to achieve one essential goal. The goal of all the paths of yoga is to be able to identify with a higher and more eternal reality as your true nature than the one you are accustomed to identify with. Once we realize that we are not our bodies nor our thinking minds or personalities we can begin to live with more peace and less fear which is the ultimate marker for advancement on the yoga path.

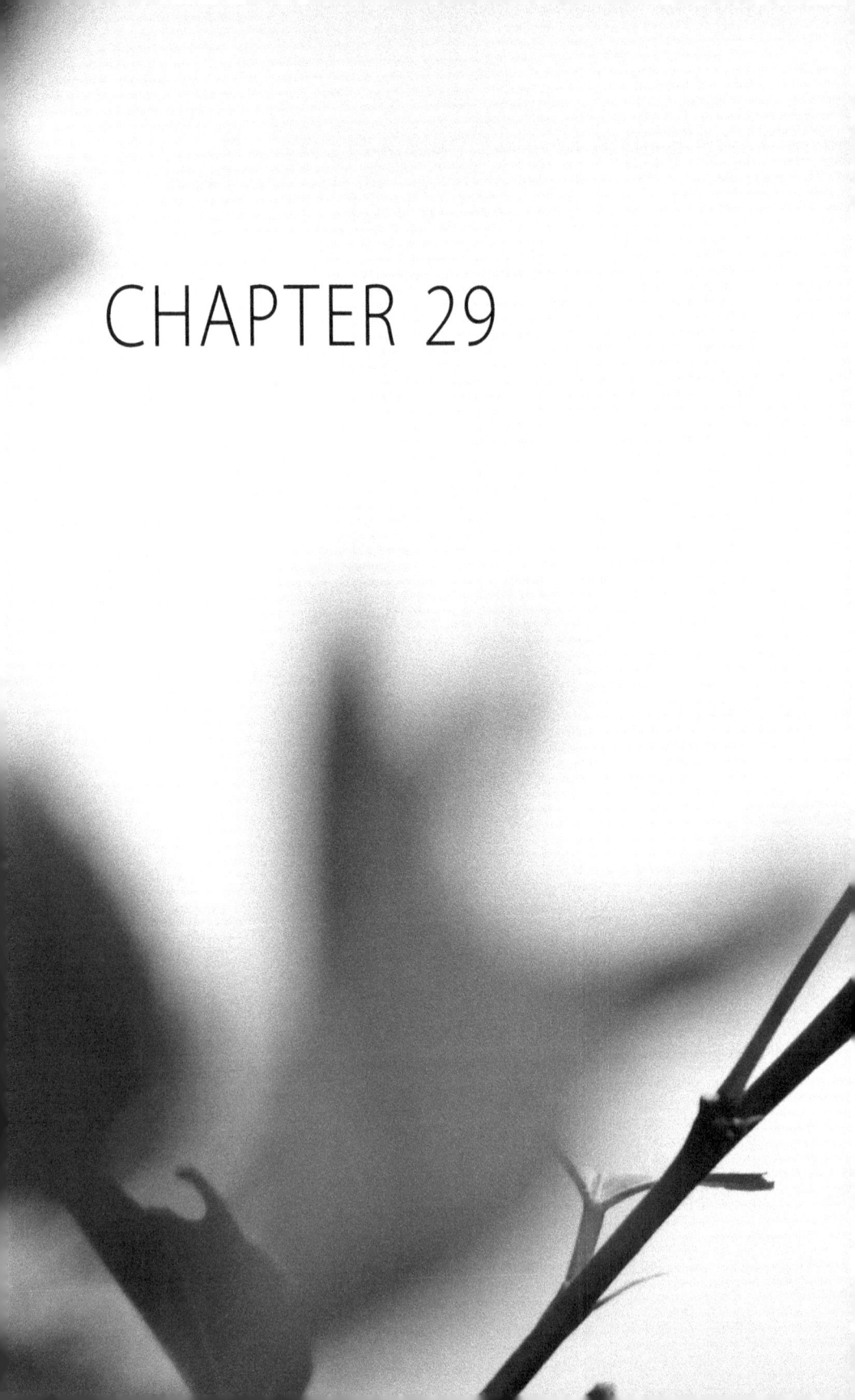

CHAPTER 29

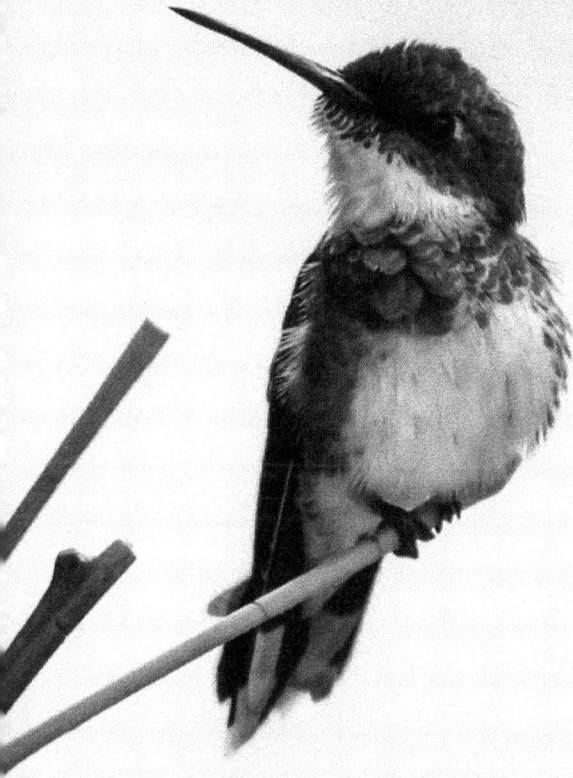

Environmental Factors and Living Organically

Living in the modern world does not make it easy to be healthy. Every day, we are exposed to a barrage of man-made environmental toxins and chemicals that invade our bodies and do harm.

Many harmful chemicals have been identified, e.g. asbestos, and have been banned and therefore the damage caused by these chemicals has been minimized. Unfortunately however people nowadays are being exposed to a vast variety of harmful chemicals that are presented as safe but are far from. In fact many if not most common chemicals used in consumer products have not been tested properly and are being used in excess by the population.

We are essentially bombarded from all different directions by poisons and toxins that are able to enter our bodies from several different ways. It is truly daunting to consider how many unnatural and thus toxic compounds and materials we are all exposed to every day. Remember that anything that enters the body that is not a food is toxic to the body, with almost no exceptions.

Perfumes and deodorants are particularly noxious even though they are commonly accepted and used by almost everyone on their skin. Mass-produced cleaning products and air fresheners also offer good examples of constant exposure to very dangerous poisons that enter our blood directly through our skin. The skin acts like a sponge absorbing into the bloodstream anything that touches it. A very good wisdom says, *if you would not eat it then do not put it on your skin*.

The family of chemicals related to sodium lauryl sulfate is another good example of a pervasive and extremely harmful molecule that even most mainstream researchers agree is dangerous to humans. Yet these chemicals are cheap to produce and thus highly profitable and so continue to be used and sold in almost every shampoo and hand soap on the market today.

The danger of these chemicals cannot be overstated.

While it may not be possible to live a life free of exposure to these environmental poisons and toxins, every bit counts as our body functions best when not bombarded by foreign chemicals. Any amount of reduction of exposure to toxins and poisons will help your body heal itself and maintain health. The human body is capable of Herculean levels of tolerance and so any percentage of help you can provide will go a long way to a stronger immune system and health.

Microfibers everywhere – Another good example of products we all assume to be safe but are not are the many different kinds of artificial fibers that we wear or sleep in. For example, nylon and spandex and microfiber sheets and clothing all rub against the skin and degrade. The skin then absorbs the microscopic particles which are harmful to the internal functioning of the body. The body does not like to be invaded by foreign materials as they are toxic.

Plastic water bottles – Perhaps most readers are familiar with the small continents of plastic garbage growing where ocean currents converge. But not only is plastic accumulating on a macro scale that we can see, rather it is even more dire when we look at the microscopic levels. Plastic is working its way up the food chain. One way we can help this is by not buying water in plastic bottles but instead to filter our own water and not using single use plastic products. This affords a very significant health benefit also because the plastic bottles break down and the toxic molecules become absorbed into the water and food consumed. Glass jars are best for water and juice!

Clean air – Many people do not have a choice as to where they live. But, within reason, we should all do our best to live in places where the air quality is not severely compromised. Cities like Los Angeles and many Chinese and Indian cities are so choked by smog that breathing is significantly compromised. Air quality is vital to the human organism and its ability to heal and maintain health.

Inside air in office buildings and even homes can be extremely polluted. Sometimes the air quality inside is even worse than the air outside, even in fairly polluted areas. We must all do our best to limit indoor air pollution. As mentioned cleaning products, sprays, and chemicals that make the air smell 'better' are never good for us. If we want to make an environment smell better it is best to use essential oil diffusers.

Clean water – The quality of our water has been damaged by human pollution and industrial indifference. Clean water is not easy to find. But once again a person simply must do their best and find the best water sources available given our location and resources. Also please be aware that the best water on earth is the water that comes inside of a fruit. Fresh fruits contain the highest quality, cleanest and most energetically charged water on earth.

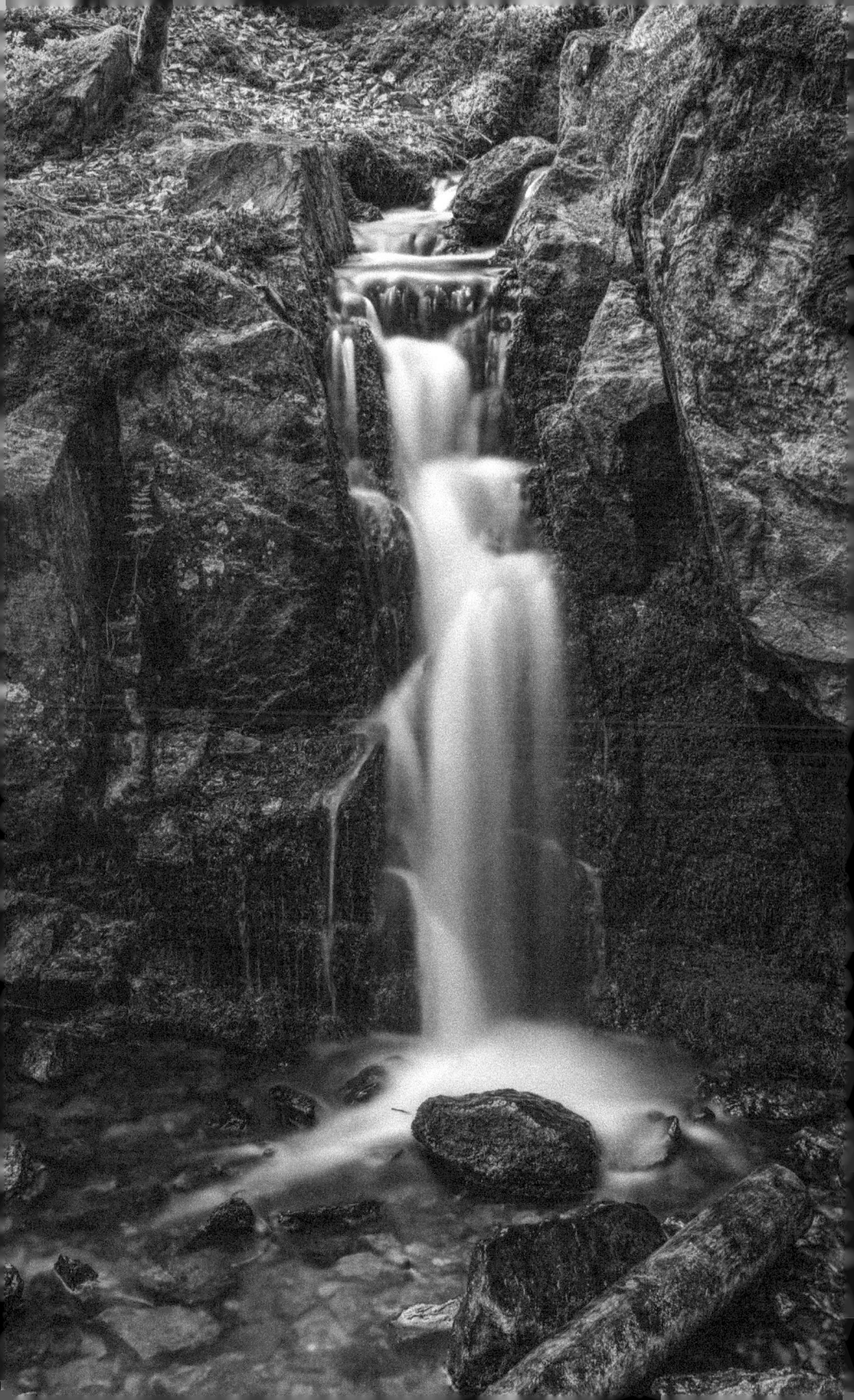

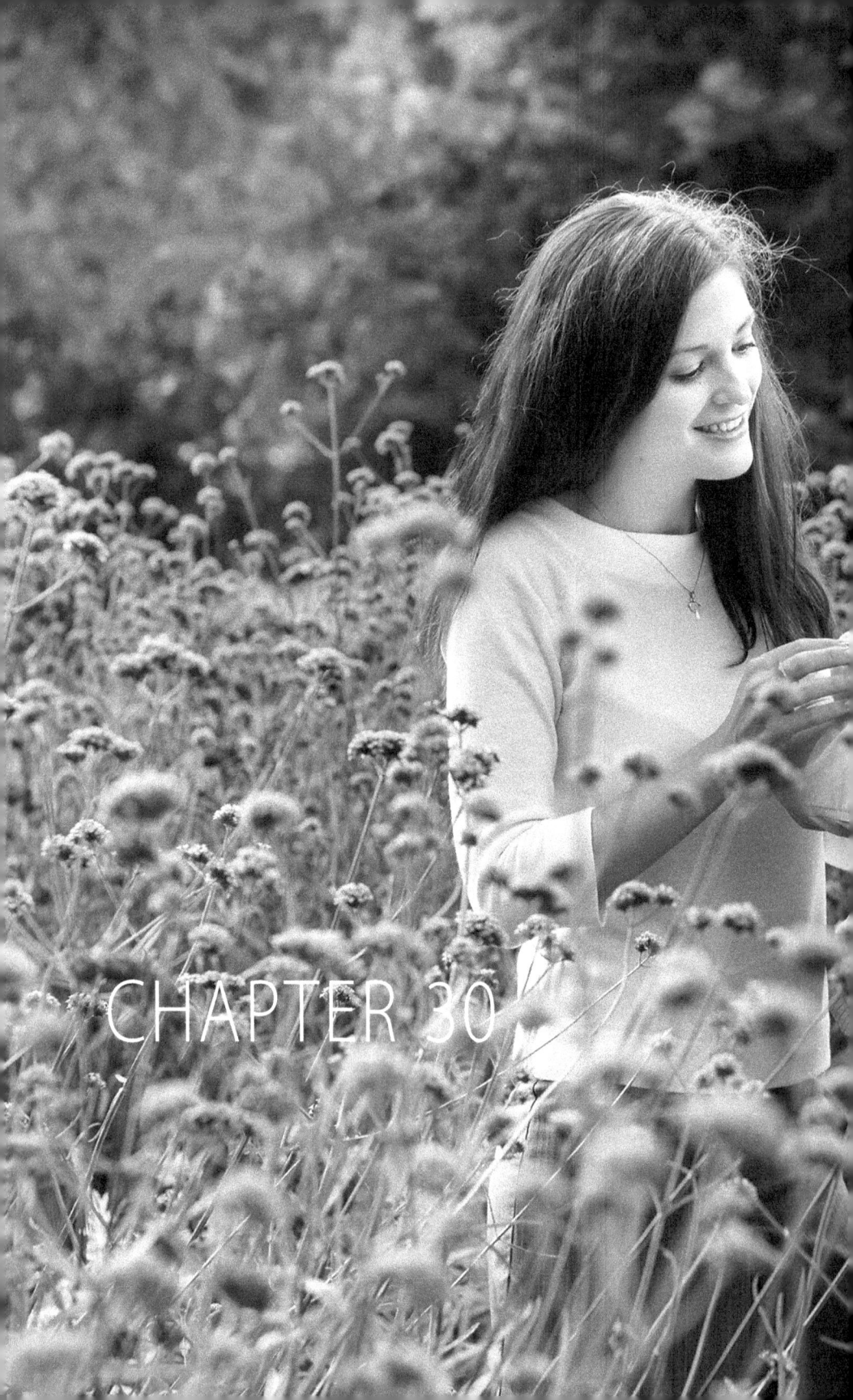

CHAPTER 30

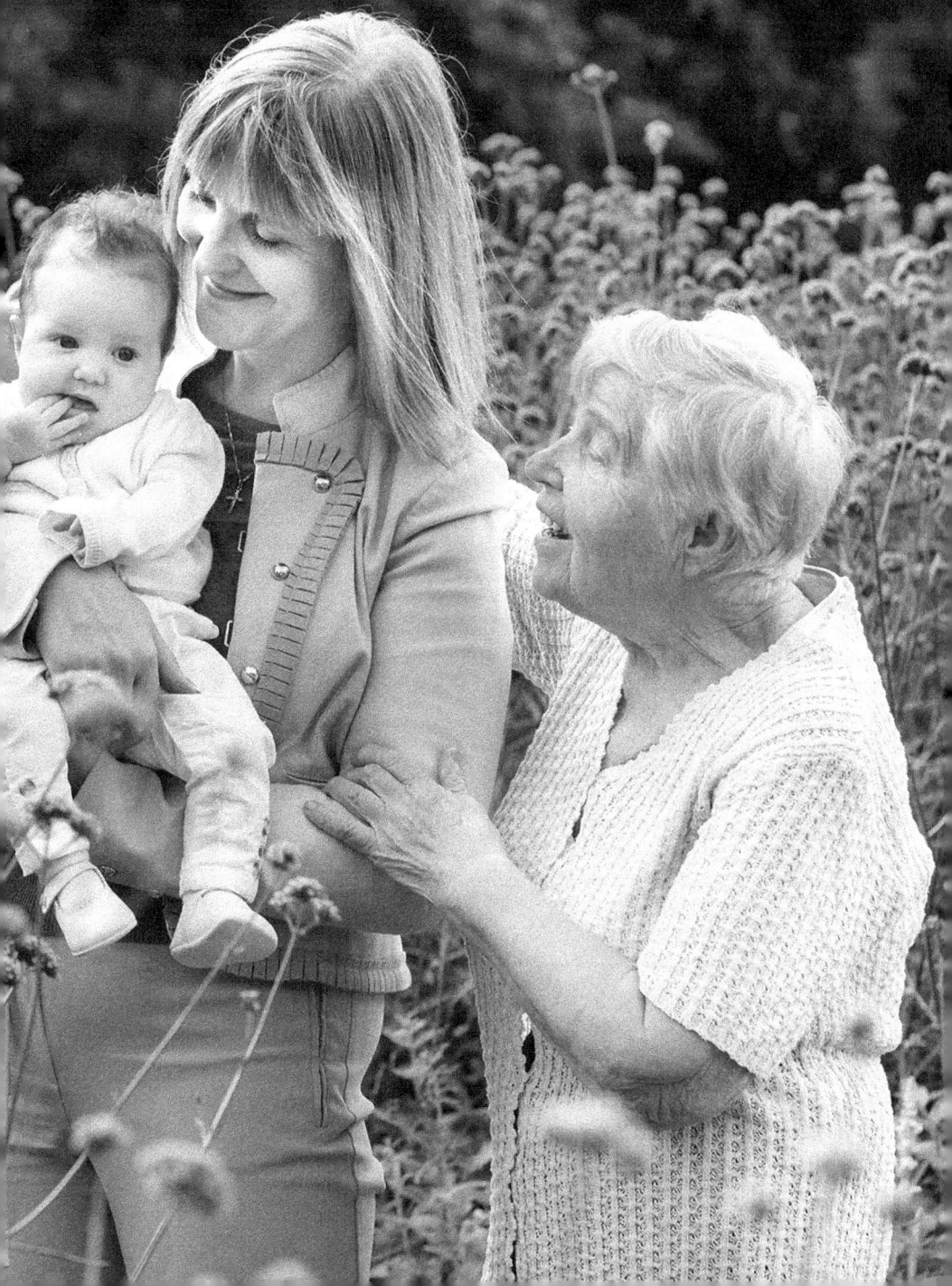

Genetics

A common set of questions goes like this from people who wonder why some people do live a long life despite poor lifestyle:

So why are lifestyle suggestions like those presented in this book important when I have an uncle who lived until he was 98 years old and he smoked cigars, drank alcohol and ate meat every day? How was my uncle able to live such a long life despite such a toxic lifestyle?

The answer is that your old uncle was born genetically stronger and more resilient than people born in subsequent decades. A person born in 1920 was born during a time in history when there were very few chemicals in the world. Therefore the mother of a person born in 1920 was not exposed to substantial levels of toxins during her pregnancy.

Unfortunately, during the last 50 years our environment has been contaminated by the innumerable pollutants we have previously discussed. This situation has led to unhealthy mothers who have an unhealthy and highly acidic gestation environment for their future babies. It is almost unimaginable the amount of chemicals and pollutants and poisons that modern humans are exposed to everyday which find their way to the fluids surrounding the fetus.

As a result, the modern woman's womb is a much less safe environment for a developing fetus. The amount of stress and damage that these toxins inflict on the genetic integrity of the baby is significant and the ensuing genetic damage can result in disease processes. Society is presently seeing this unfortunate trend manifest the disturbing prevalence of childhood cancers and other severe diseases that are common today in children. Any time a child has a serious disease it is a function of weak genetics and/or exposure to toxins...which often as we just described are related.

Everybody has different genetics. After following the same poor lifestyle, Person A may get diabetes while Person B may develop hypertension while Person C may get some type of cancer. In none of these cases would the person have developed those conditions had they followed a lifestyle in line with their biology.

Do not ever fear getting the same disease as your parents unless you live in a way that puts pressure on your genetics the same as they did. The idea of genetic predetermination does not hold true unless the same lifestyle pressures are applied to the next generation.

In sum, to protect the lives of our generation and of future generations we must simply clean up our act. Failure must not be an option. And every small reduction in toxic exposure goes a long way.

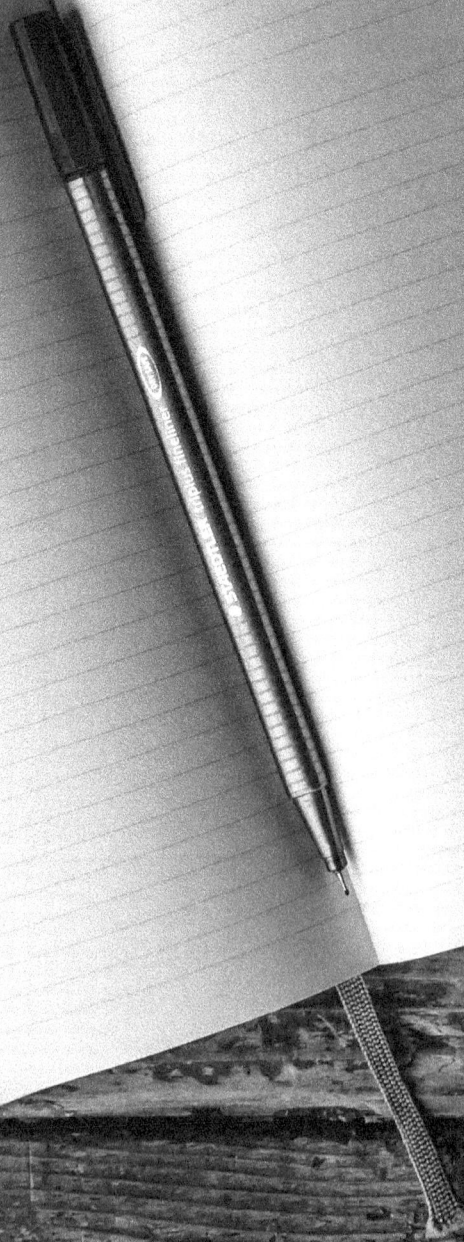

CHAPTER 31

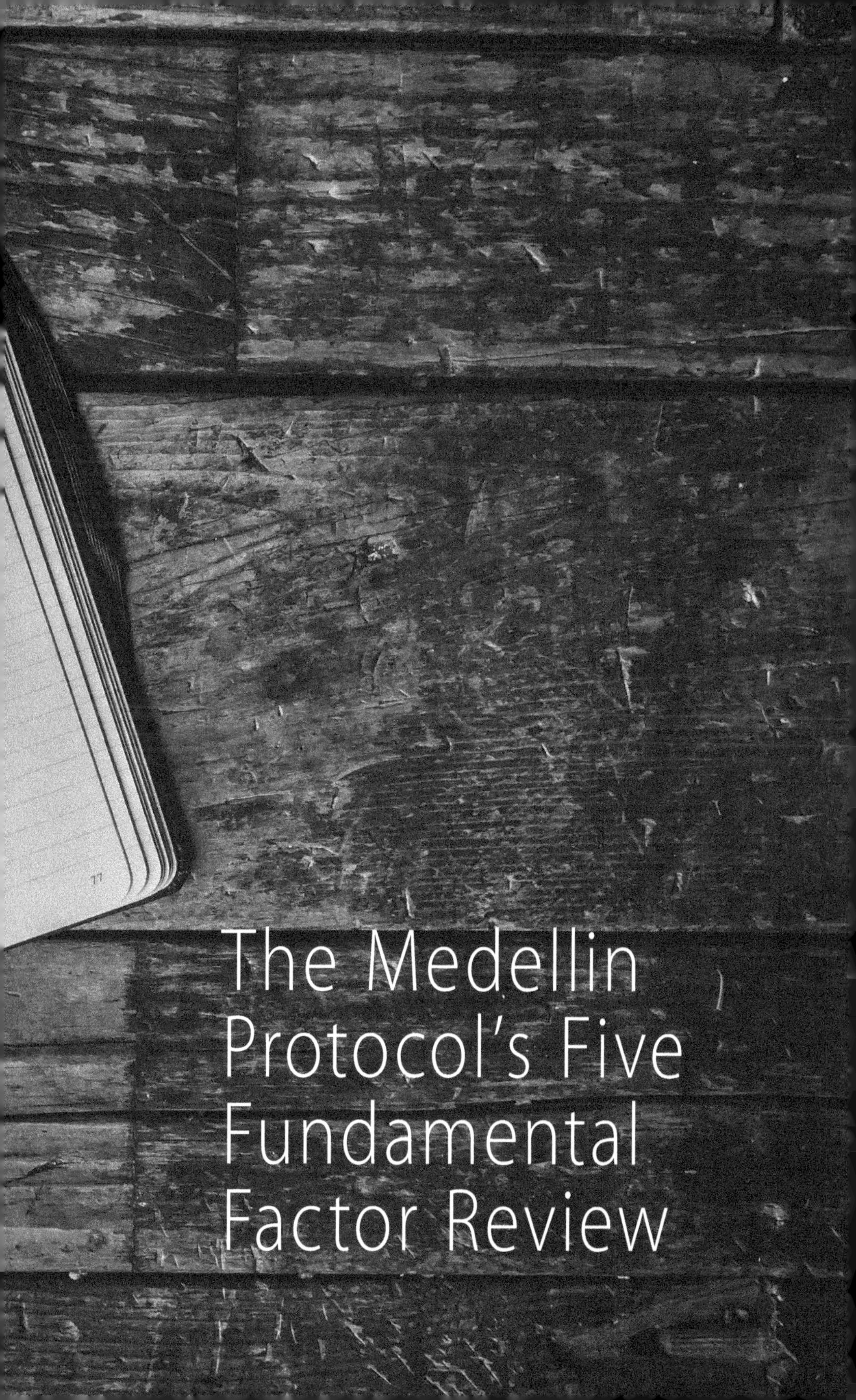

The Medellin Protocol's Five Fundamental Factor Review

To review, applying the Five Fundamental Factors will be the foundation of the path towards healing and wellbeing.

1. How Do We Eat?

   Eat as much fruit as possible and no animal products.

2. How Do We Exercise?

   Yoga is ideal and all exercise is good! Every day is best!

3. How Do We Think?

   Awareness and mind – practice meditation.

4. How Do We Rest?

   Rest and sleep must not be compromised if possible.

5. How Do We Live More Organically?

   Limit environmental toxin exposure as much as possible.

As you now understand, these Five Fundamental Factors of the Medellin Protocol as practiced at the Medellin Wellness Center in Colombia form the variables of an equation that when aligned to biology deliver a stronger immune system and greater health in almost all cases.

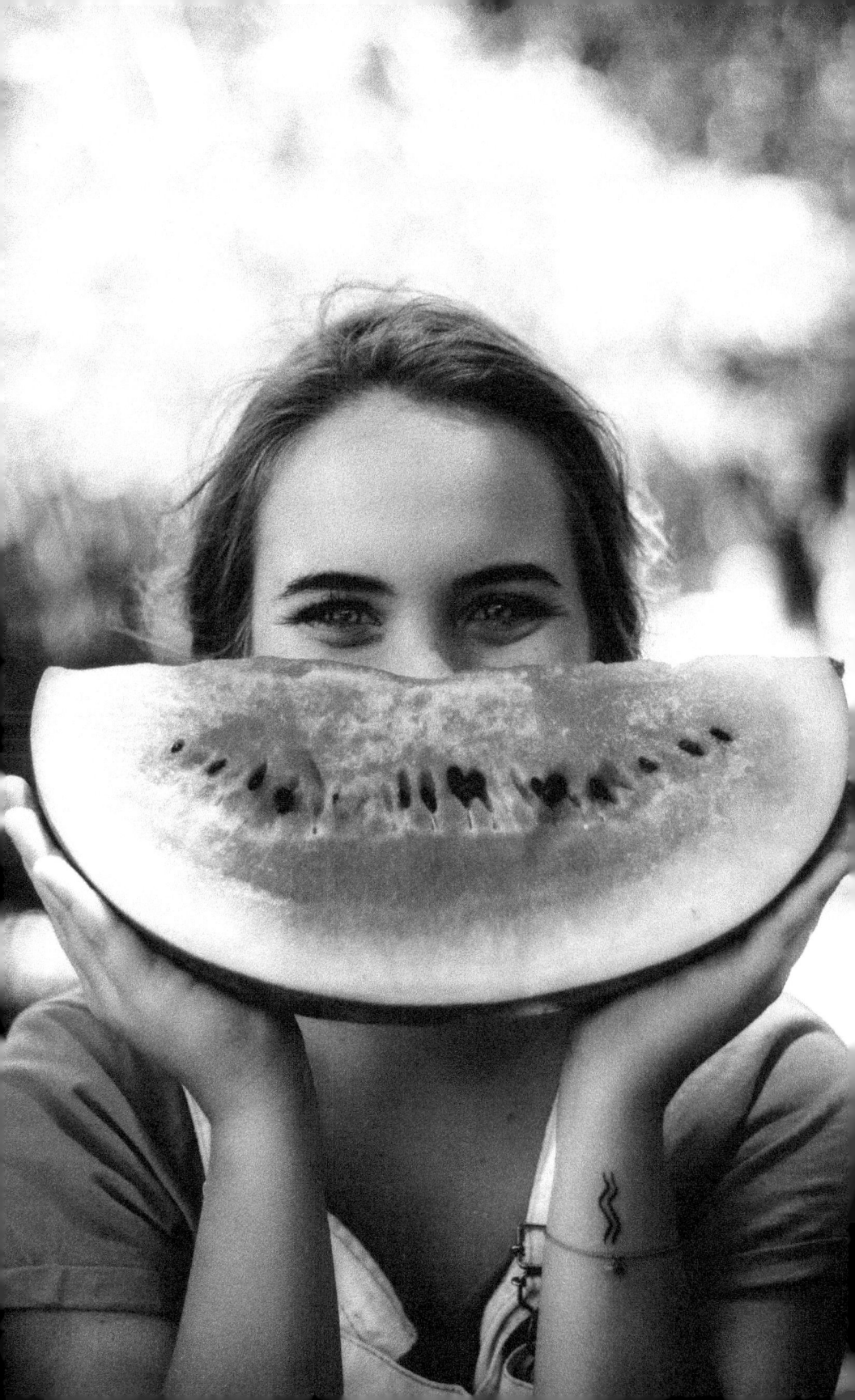

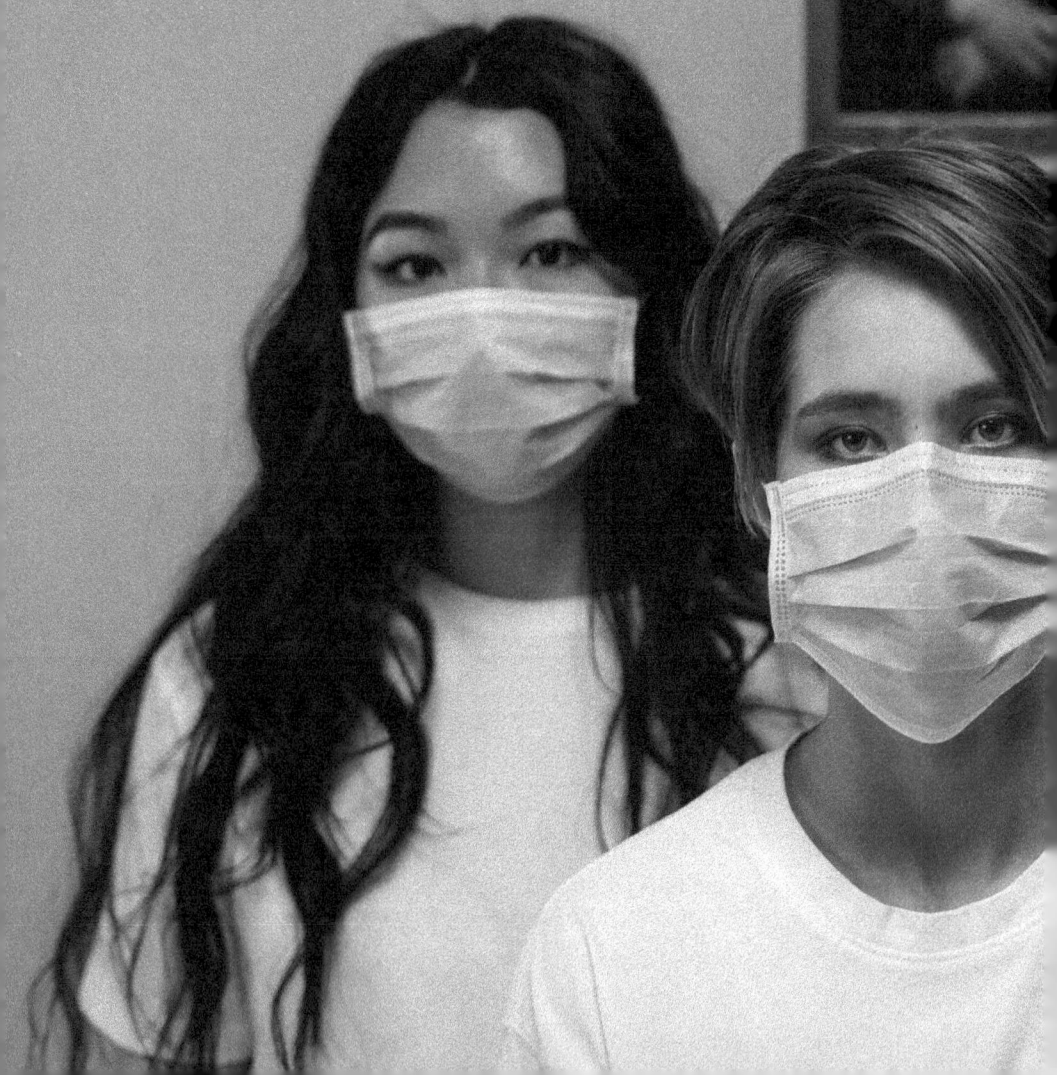

Chapter 32

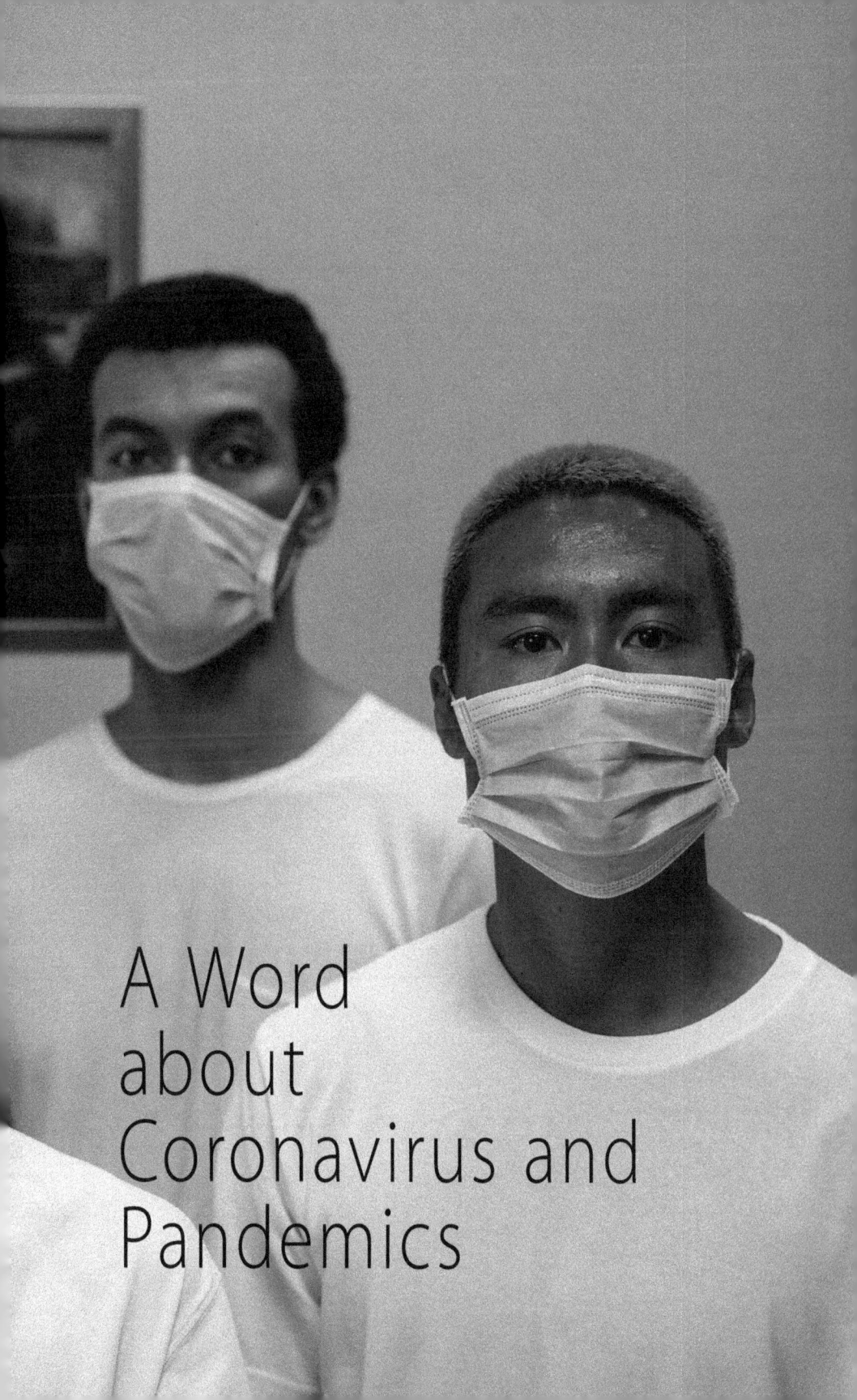

A Word
about
Coronavirus and
Pandemics

The catastrophic effect of the 2019/20 pandemic upon the health and economic wellbeing of our planet brings into sharp focus the vital importance of our immune system to protect us.

What is clear to all who observe is that the health of a person's immune system is the key factor in determining the effect of the pandemic on those who are exposed.

Those who have impaired immune systems related to underlying health conditions such as diabetes, obesity, high blood pressure, cancer, pulmonary and cardiac diseases and other conditions are much more likely to become extremely ill or die.

Those who have healthy immune systems are much more likely to experience mild symptoms or in many cases remain completely asymptomatic.

Because the Five Fundamental Factors of the Medellin Wellness Protocol are specifically designed to promote the most important elements that strengthen our immune system, the Medellin Wellness Protocol can become a powerful weapon against any disease including pandemics.

Pandemics will continue to spread on earth to the combination of animal exploitation and human density and as a result the only solution is to have the healthiest immune system possible and then to not live in fear.

From the Author

As we face unprecedented times and challenges on this planet it becomes more important than ever to understand the fundamental factors presented in this book that build resilience of body and mind.

I wrote this book for the general public because I strongly believe that everyone should learn this information. Once the information is learned people are welcome to do whatever they wish including incorporating it into their life or not.

I often recite the famous quote that 'knowledge is power' and it is my position that the main reason why people do not eat smarter, or exercise more, or use their mind in negative ways, or expose themselves to toxins without knowing, is lack of information.

My experience in the field of wellness and nutrition over the last twenty years has taught me that when people learn about the facts of biology and anatomy it is much easier if not almost effortless to transition to a different way of eating.

I have also seen that after as little as four weeks of eating better and applying the factors discussed in this book that students relate experiences and benefits that are remarkable and this provides them the motivation needed to keep going and feel even stronger.

It is my hope and prayer that the information in this book will inspire the reader to do what must be done to achieve optimal health in all dimensions and to live a life without fear.

Fred

www.ingramcontent.com/pod-product-compliance
Lightning Source LLC
Chambersburg PA
CBHW051439270326
41931CB00020B/3477